ANTI INFLAMMATORY COOKBOOK

For Family

100+ meticulously crafted recipes, meticulously curated and endorsed by pediatricians, offering an impeccable pathway to revolutionize your family's well-being.

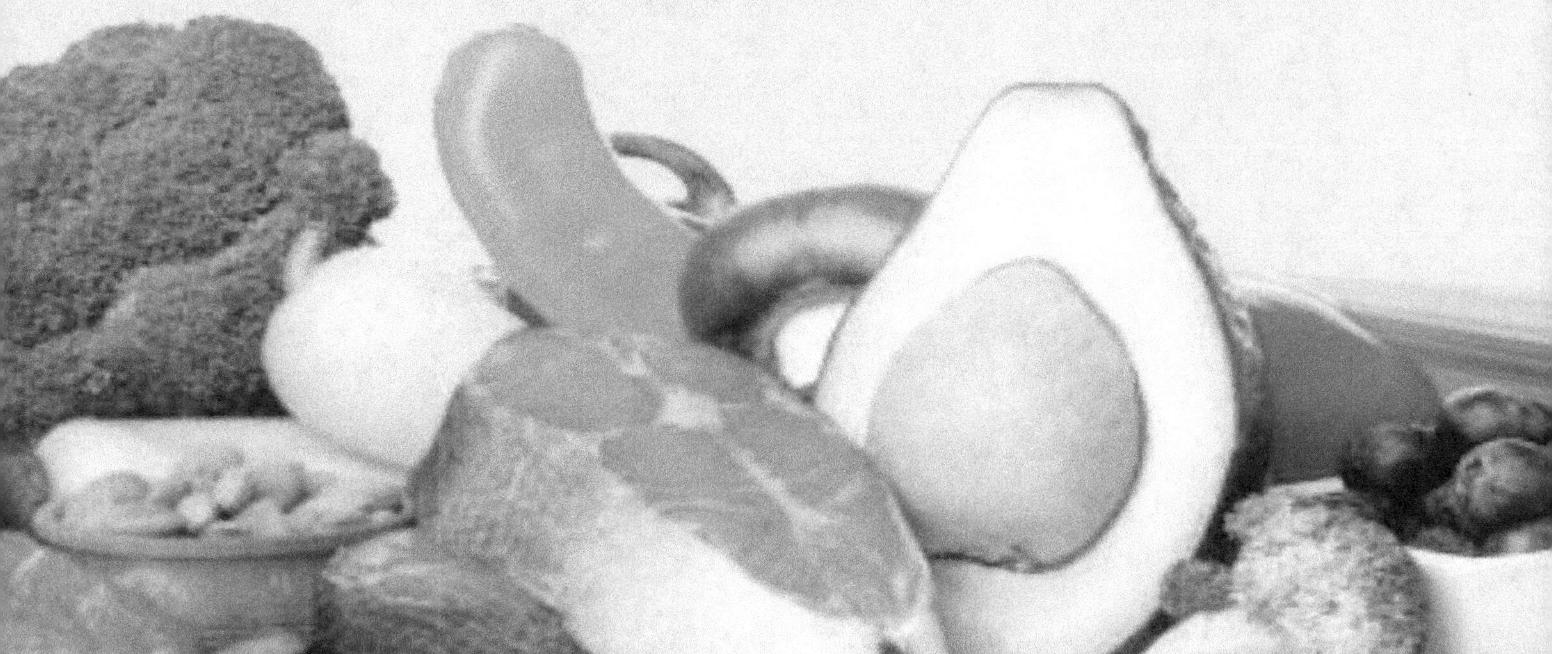

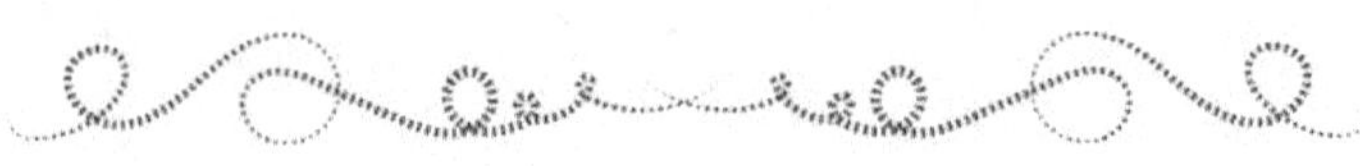

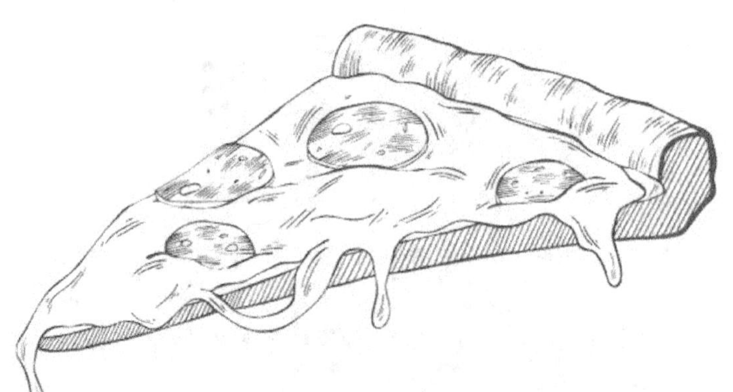

Copyright © 2024 VIVIAN GREENE

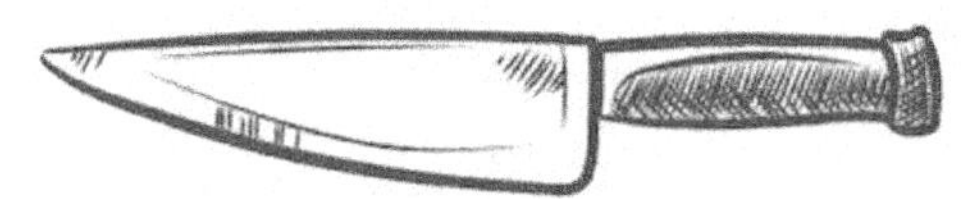

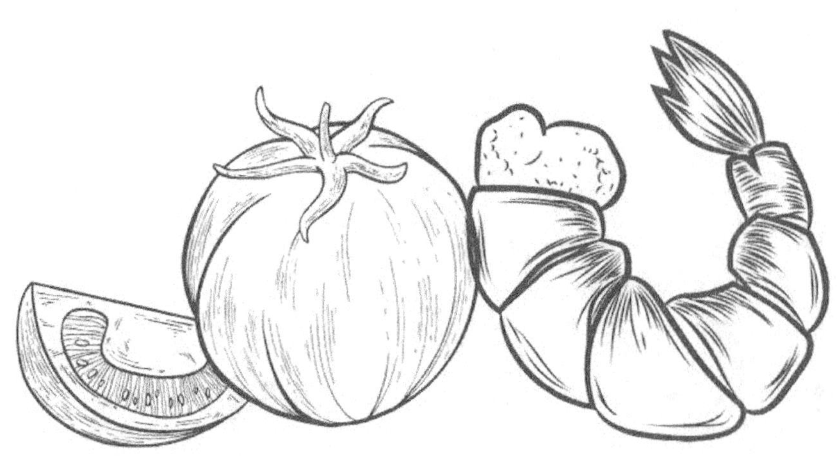

TABLE OF CONTENTS

Introduction

Nowadays, when people are more aware of their health than ever, pursuing well-being has become a daily priority. The power of anti-inflammatory living is one idea that sticks out among the multitude of dietary methods as a beacon of holistic health. Introducing the "Anti-Anti-Inflammatory Cookbook for Family," a culinary adventure that embraces an anti-inflammatory lifestyle to transform your family's health.

Once thought to be the body's normal reaction to damage or illness, inflammation has become a crucial topic in the field of health and wellbeing. Acute inflammation serves as a protective, limited reaction, but persistent inflammation is a hidden cause of several health issues. This low-grade, chronic inflammation affects not just the health of individuals but also the vitality of whole families and is linked to ailments ranging from autoimmune disorders to cardiovascular diseases.

But worry not—the "Anti-Anti-Inflammatory" method, a paradigm shift, is hidden inside the pages of this cookbook. Our culinary philosophy aims to actively combat the consequences of inflammation through a carefully chosen array of dishes, rather than just negating it. We provide a symphony of tastes that are intended to not only entice the senses but also to feed and cure the body from the inside out, taking inspiration from an abundance of healthful products.

The days of connecting nutritious eating to starvation or bland food are long gone. The "Anti-Anti-Inflammatory Cookbook" is a celebration of inventive cooking that demonstrates that tasty does not have to equate to healthful. Every dish is an ode to the harmonic union of flavor and health, offering your family not only a culinary feast but also support on their path to better health.

Every recipe in these pages has been painstakingly created and approved by doctors as part of our commitment to quality. We work with medical professionals to guarantee that every meal complies with the highest standards of health and wellness since we understand the specific nutritional requirements of families, particularly those with young children.

Think of this cookbook as your road map for changing your family's health trajectory as you set out on this culinary journey. Come along as we redefine health, one delicious dish at a time. Let the "Anti-Anti-Inflammatory Cookbook for Family" serve as your guide to a future in which health is a way of life rather than merely a destination.

Cheers to thriving health, wholesome food, and the anti-inflammatory effect that may change lives!

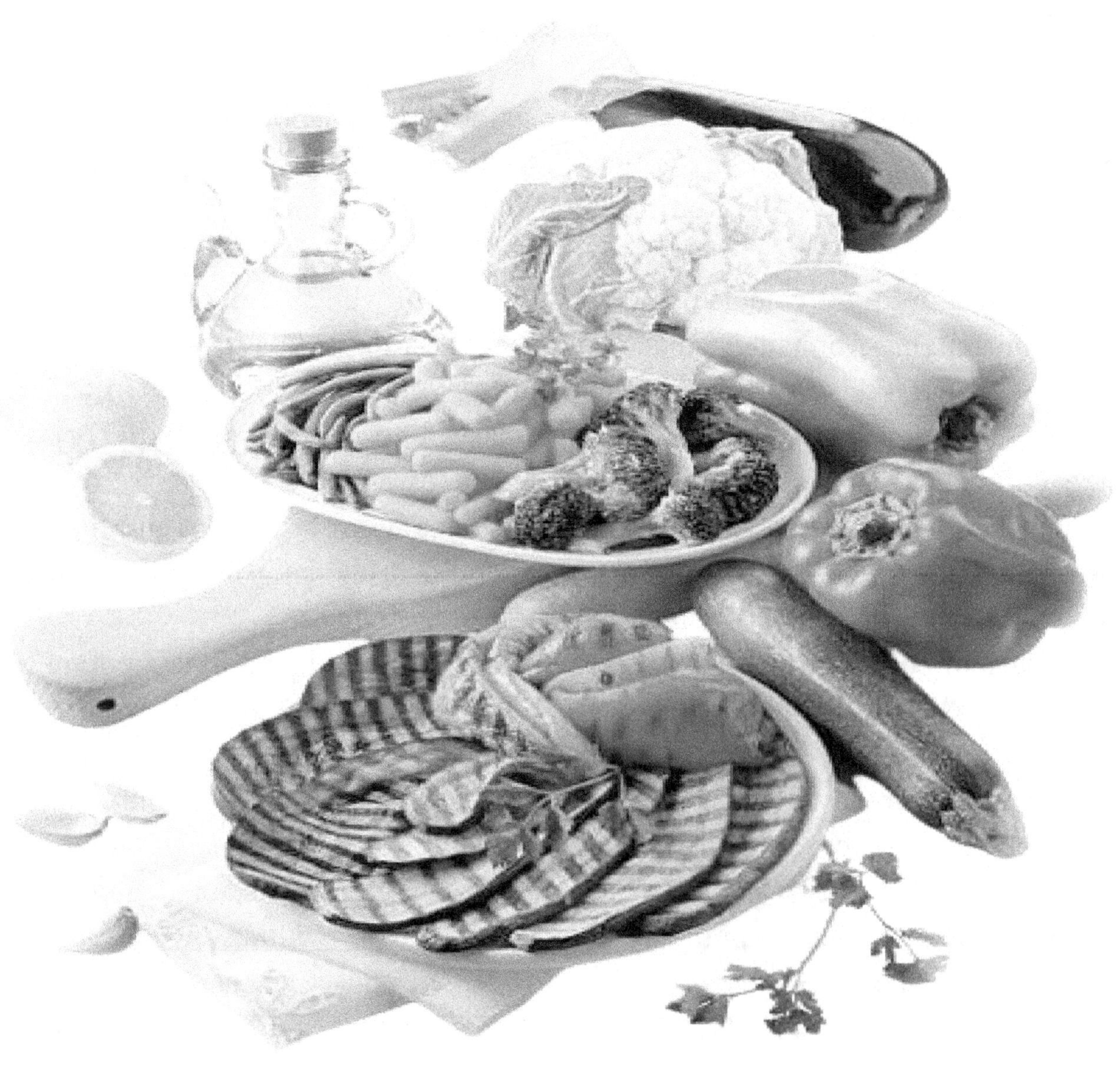

Within the field of modern health and nutrition sciences, inflammation has emerged as a key element affecting general health and well-being. Among the plethora of dietary theories, the Anti-Anti-Inflammatory approach stands out as a strategic paradigm intended to address the complex relationship between inflammation and food rather than just a fad. This method actively uses diet to promote optimum health while simultaneously attempting to lessen the negative consequences of chronic inflammation. The following are the main arguments in favor of an anti-inflammatory strategy when aiming for overall well-being.

1. Addressing Chronic Inflammation, the Silent Culprit
Chronic inflammation, which is often subtle and unnoticeable, has been linked to a wide range of illnesses, including autoimmune disorders and cardiovascular ailments. In contrast to acute inflammation, which is the body's normal, localized reaction to damage, chronic inflammation may last for long periods and aggravate overall health issues. The Anti-Anti-Inflammatory method uses a sophisticated understanding of the link between dietary choices and inflammation to acknowledge the need to treat this hidden culprit thoroughly.

2. Comprehensive Wellbeing Exceeding Symptom Handling
The Anti-Anti-Inflammatory paradigm takes a more comprehensive approach, while conventional anti-inflammatory methods can concentrate on symptom treatment. It aims to produce an environment in the body that actively counteracts inflammatory processes, as opposed to only decreasing inflammation reactively. Through using the innate anti-inflammatory characteristics of well-chosen meals, this method seeks to foster a long-lasting feeling of well-being, beyond the constraints of treatment-focused approaches.

3. Family Well-Being-Endorsed Precision by Pediatricians

Importantly, the anti-inflammatory method is a precision-guided tactic rather than a one-size-fits-all one, which is particularly important for families. Pediatricians support this method because it acknowledges that each person has varied dietary demands at various stages of life and makes sure that all recipes meet the highest standards of safety and effectiveness. The Anti-Anti-Inflammatory Cookbook becomes a reliable ally in promoting the health of the whole family by combining professional ideas.

4. Gastronomic Delight without Sacrifice
Unlike popular belief, which links healthy eating to strict cooking, the Anti-Anti-Inflammatory method honors the union of taste and nutrition. It demonstrates how well-thought-out recipe creation can make healthy meals decadent, interesting, and enjoyable. This reworking of the story around food is a statement that health should be a fulfilling journey rather than a sacrifice, in addition to encouraging people to make better decisions.

5. Encouraging People to Take Charge of Their Health
In the end, the Anti-Anti-Inflammatory method gives people the ability to take charge of their health. It offers a useful road map for anyone looking to make well-informed nutritional decisions by providing a well-selected assortment of recipes. Families and individuals may both take proactive measures to strengthen their well-being and develop a sustainable, health-conscious lifestyle by adopting this strategy.
 The Anti-Anti-Inflammatory method is a calculated reaction to the many problems that chronic inflammation presents, rather than just a dietary philosophy. Based on scientific knowledge, doctor support, and deliciousness, it serves as a lighthouse pointing people in the direction of a time when well-being is a concrete, long-term reality rather than just an ideal.

Beyond recipes, the "Anti-Anti-Inflammatory Cookbook" proves to be a transformational instrument in the search for a healthier and more lively family life. This recipe book is painstakingly crafted to transform your family's health by using a purposeful and holistic approach to eating. Here's how using this cookbook as a catalyst might improve your loved ones' health and happiness.

1. Encouraging Dietary Decisions

The ability to empower your family with knowledgeable healthy choices is at the heart of this cookbook. Every dish uses carefully chosen components that are well known for their anti-inflammatory qualities, making every meal a chance to strengthen one's health. Gaining knowledge about the nutritional content of the foods you eat will enable you to make decisions that are healthy for your family as a whole.

2. Diminishing Inflammatory Stress

Modern food habits often promote chronic inflammation, which may be a quiet health disruptor. This recipe offers a step-by-step guide to drastically lower the body's inflammatory burden for your family. The addition of anti-inflammatory components and the removal of possible triggers are in line with the overarching objective of creating an atmosphere that promotes long-term and optimum health.

3. Diverse Cuisines for Enjoyable Eating

Eating healthfully doesn't have to equate to boredom. The "Anti-Anti-Inflammatory Cookbook" opens your family's eyes to a world of flavorful variety where wholesome meals are a gastronomic joy. This cookbook demonstrates that health-conscious choices can live together with a rich tapestry of tastes, making every meal an occasion to cherish. It offers everything from colorful breakfast alternatives to substantial meals and delicious sweets.

4. A Shift to a Family-Centric Lifestyle

This cookbook encourages a family-oriented lifestyle transition outside of the kitchen. Your family may start a common path to well-being by accepting the anti-

anti-inflammatory concepts as a group. Cooking and dining together creates a feeling of community and purpose, which strengthens the idea that maintaining good health is a team effort woven into day-to-day existence.

5. Assurance Endorsed by Pediatricians

The support of pediatricians for this cookbook is one of its distinctive advantages. The recipes on these pages are more than simply delicious dishes; they are carefully prepared with your family's health in mind. This endorsement adds degree of comfort by guaranteeing parents that all dishes meet the strictest standards for nutritional quality and safety, which is especially important when taking into account the special requirements of developing children.

6. Long-Term Health Practices

For a change to have significance, it must be enduring. The Anti-Anti-Inflammatory Cookbook is a manual for creating long-lasting health practices in your household. By incorporating these dishes into your usual cooking routine, you're not simply starting a short-term diet; rather, you're setting the groundwork for long-term health that becomes a way of life for your family.

Essentially, the "Anti-Anti-Inflammatory Cookbook" is more than just a cookbook; it's a full manual for improving your family's health. Accepting the values in these pages means starting a journey that goes beyond the kitchen and incorporates happiness, health, and togetherness into the everyday routine of your family. This cookbook is about the transforming potential of deliberate, health-conscious living for future generations—it's not just about what you eat.

Chapter 1: Understanding Inflammation

What is Inflammation?

Within the complex web of the human body's defenses, inflammation appears as a basic and sophisticated reaction to different stimuli, indicating the body's natural capacity to defend and repair. Understanding the complexities of inflammation is essential to understanding physiological resilience, an area of great significance for individuals looking to maximize their health and well-being.

Fundamentally, inflammation is a highly controlled and dynamic biological response that happens in response to infections, injured cells, or irritants. This complex procedure sets up a series of actions intended to eradicate the pathogen and start the healing process. Fundamentally, inflammation acts as a physiological sentinel of the body's defensive systems, watching out for any dangers.

The classic signs of inflammation include redness, heat, swelling, and pain, all of which are indicative of different cellular and molecular processes occurring at the region of concern. To restore homeostasis within the injured tissue, a multitude of immune cells, signaling molecules, and metabolic pathways collaborate in this coordinated dance.

To comprehend inflammation, one must acknowledge that it is bimodal, occurring in both acute and chronic forms. One of the most important aspects of the healing process is acute inflammation, which is the body's rapid and localized reaction to injury or infection. It responds quickly and forcefully, eliminating dangers and starting the healing process for injured tissues. Within this framework, inflammation serves as a protective and beneficial mechanism, safeguarding equilibrium.

On the other hand, chronic inflammation deviates from the physiological normal and is characterized by a low-grade and persistent immune system activation. It has been identified as a key role in the etiology of a number of chronic illnesses, such as metabolic syndromes, autoimmune diseases, and cardiovascular diseases. Chronic inflammation, in contrast to its acute cousin, may persist and cause long-term tissue damage as well as problems with systemic health.

Inflammation may be caused by a variety of things, including internal dysregulation and external infections. Classical triggers include infections, injuries, and irritants; they initiate the body's defensive systems. However lifestyle variables may also contribute to the persistence of inflammation, creating a complicated interaction between internal and environmental stimuli. These include sedentary behaviors, poor food choices, and chronic stress.

A balanced approach is advocated by a comprehensive viewpoint for navigating the world of inflammation. The objective is to correctly control and end the response, even though acute inflammation is a normal and essential aspect of immunological activity. Furthermore, keeping inflammation from becoming chronic becomes essential to preserving good health.

Let us now discuss anti-inflammatory methods, which include dietary habits, lifestyle choices, and wellness practices designed to reduce the body's inflammatory load. A diet high in items that reduce inflammation, such as fruits, vegetables, nuts, and fatty fish, becomes essential to this effort. Reducing stress, getting enough sleep, and engaging in physical exercise all help to create an atmosphere that is favorable to reducing inflammation.

Inflammation is a complicated and multifaceted physiological reaction that plays a dual role in the development of health and illness. A basic comprehension of its dynamics enables people to make well-informed decisions about acute conditions as well as the development of a lifestyle that reduces the likelihood of chronic inflammatory disorders. By using this perspective, inflammation is no longer seen as a mystery force but rather as a part of our biological resilience that may lead to long-term health and well-being if it is recognized and understood.

It is critical to comprehend the deep effects of inflammation on the complex fabric of family health. Inflammation, especially in its chronic form, is no longer just associated with damage and infection. It now plays a complex role in the larger picture of well-being. In this thorough investigation, we explore the nuances of how inflammation may profoundly impact the dynamics of health within a family.

The Inflammatory Process's Biological Roots

Let's first understand the basic underpinnings of inflammation before we can fully understand its influence. When inflammation is present in an acute state, the body responds naturally and locally, acting as an evolutionary defensive mechanism to keep the body safe. But when inflammation lasts for an extended period, the story changes completely. It is now known that several different health disorders are significantly influenced by this protracted inflammatory state, which is often subtle and sneaky.

In a time when heart health is vital, the development and progression of cardiovascular disorders have been linked to chronic inflammation, which is a depressing fact. The inflammatory response raises the risk of heart attacks and strokes by impairing blood flow and facilitating the development of arterial plaque. This means that families will be more aware of the food and lifestyle choices that either exacerbate or reduce inflammation.

Effects on the Immune System

The inflammatory response is closely linked to the immune system, which is the guardian of our well-being. Prolonged inflammation may weaken the immune system, making a person more vulnerable to infections and requiring more time to heal. In a family setting, this entails realizing that lifestyle decisions and everyday decisions made in the kitchen have an impact on the household's overall immunological resilience.

The relationship between brain health and chronic inflammation has been clarified by recent studies. Cognitive deficits and diseases like Alzheimer's disease have been linked to inflammation in the brain. The ramifications for family health are significant, and this calls for a more thorough investigation of food habits that either reduce or increase inflammation in the complex web of brain connections.

Joint and Muscle-Related Issues

It is impossible to overestimate the effect of inflammation on joint and musculoskeletal health in families with different age groups. Chronic inflammation may affect mobility and general quality of life, and it can be a contributing factor to illnesses like arthritis. Families take proactive steps, putting nutrition at the top of the list, after realizing the impact inflammation plays in many ailments.

The younger family members are also affected by inflammation. Pediatricians are realizing that early dietary habits may determine long-term health, which is why they are emphasizing the importance of food in children's health. In youngsters, chronic inflammation has been linked to allergies, asthma, and even behavioral problems. As a result, the family kitchen becomes an important setting for determining the next generation's health trajectory.

Knowing how inflammation affects family health should not be a reason for despair but rather for action. Families are encouraged to adopt an Anti-Anti-Inflammatory strategy, which is a proactive approach aimed at reducing inflammation via well-informed food decisions. With the help of anti-inflammatory foods and reducing possible triggers, families may take a group trip toward improved health.

The keystone of this educational project is empowerment. Armed with information, families take control of their health, avoiding trigger points and moving in the direction of long-term, sustainable well-being. Beyond theory, this teaching reaches into the real world, where everyday choices made in the kitchen may effectively reduce inflammation and promote a strong family health paradigm.

 The investigation of inflammation's effects on family health is complex and encompasses aspects of immunological response, neurological health, musculoskeletal durability, cardiovascular health, and pediatric concerns. Families who comprehend these nuances are better able to make choices that go beyond personal health and help to create a robust, anti-inflammatory fabric of well-being for future generations.

The Anti-Anti-Inflammatory diet is more than just a food fad; it's a shining star in the always-changing field of dietary philosophies. Based on a deep knowledge of the effects of inflammation on health, this dietary strategy provides a range of advantages that go far beyond personal health. Here, we share the game-changing benefits of adopting an anti-inflammatory diet.

1. Reducing Long-Term Inflammation

The main goal of the anti-inflammatory diet is to reduce chronic inflammation, which is at its core. People actively combat the systemic inflammation that may lead to a variety of health problems by choosing meals high in anti-inflammatory qualities. This proactive approach turns into a pillar in the care and prevention of ailments ranging from autoimmune illnesses to cardiovascular problems.

2. Resilience in Cardiology

The beneficial effects of this dietary paradigm on cardiovascular health are among its most notable advantages. Including foods high in heart-healthy fats, antioxidants, and anti-inflammatory properties helps to maintain healthy cholesterol levels, minimize the risk of arterial plaque development, and promote optimum blood vessel function. A stronger cardiovascular system that encourages lifespan and vigor is the end outcome.

3. Enhanced Immunity

A diet high in anti-inflammatory foods strengthens the immune system. Through the consumption of nutrient-dense, anti-inflammatory meals, people create an environment in their bodies that promotes strong immunity. In addition to lowering vulnerability to infections, this promotes general resistance against microbial challenges by enabling a quicker recovery when disease occurs.

4. Health of the Nerves

The Anti-Anti-Inflammatory diet takes seriously the complex link that is emerging between nutrition and neurological health. This dietary strategy, which includes foods high in antioxidants and neuroprotective chemicals, is linked to a lower risk of neurodegenerative diseases. Potential advantages include improved emotional control, cognitive performance, and general brain health.

5. Musculoskeletal and Joint Health

An encouraging development for those suffering from musculoskeletal problems and joint discomfort is the Anti-Anti-Inflammatory diet. Some of the items in this diet have anti-inflammatory qualities that may help reduce arthritis-related symptoms. People may improve general mobility, lower inflammation, and promote joint health by actively adopting these foods.

6. Control of Weight

An anti-inflammatory diet has the natural side effect of helping people lose weight. Those who choose nutrient-dense, whole meals often find it simpler to keep their weight in check. This dietary strategy inhibits the ingestion of processed, inflammatory foods that lead to weight gain and, as a result, a host of health problems related to obesity.

7. Health of Children

The Anti-Anti-Inflammatory diet's versatility for a range of age groups, including kids, is a benefit that is often ignored. Including healthy, anti-inflammatory foods in family meals helps the youngest members build a foundation for lifetime health. This dietary strategy is recommended by pediatricians because it may have a good effect on children's development and reduce the likelihood of inflammatory problems in children.

8. Transition to a Sustainable Lifestyle

In contrast to fad diets that guarantee instant results, the Anti-Anti-Inflammatory diet promotes a long-term lifestyle change. A long-term commitment to making health-conscious decisions is more likely to be embraced when people are encouraged to adore eating wholesome, tasty meals. Because of their durability, the advantages last longer than fleeting enhancements and integrate into a more comprehensive, health-conscious way of living.

The foods that are recommended in an anti-inflammatory diet also provide a wide range of advantages. This nutritional strategy goes beyond being just a fad and does more than just reduce chronic inflammation. It also strengthens cardiovascular health, boosts immunity, and promotes general well-being. It turns into a life-changing path towards long-term health, a comprehensive model that gives people the ability to take control of their vitality and rewrite the story of their wellbeing.

Chapter 2: Building a Foundation

Stocking a Healthy Kitchen

Maintaining a wholesome kitchen is the first step in developing a healthy lifestyle. Start with an abundance of fresh fruits and vegetables, which are colorful providers of vital vitamins and antioxidants. Sustained energy and fiber are provided by whole grains like quinoa, brown rice, and oats, while lean proteins like chicken, fish, and legumes serve as the building blocks for healthy muscles. Cardiovascular health is enhanced by essential fats found in foods like avocados, almonds, and olive oil.

Choose whole-grain bread and pasta instead of refined sugars, and replace artificial sweeteners with natural ones like honey or maple syrup. Spices and herbs give a taste without adding extra sugar or salt, and they also have anti-inflammatory qualities. Maintain a well-hydrated home by consuming a lot of water and herbal teas while avoiding sugar-filled drinks. Establishing a kitchen filled with healthy alternatives makes your home an easily accessible sanctuary for health-conscious decisions, facilitating your family's path toward vitality and overall well-being.

Essential Ingredients

When it comes to the Anti-Anti-Inflammatory diet, the key to great cooking is the thoughtful selection of key components. These components serve as the foundation for delectable meals but also have transforming properties that actively reduce chronic inflammation and advance general well-being.

1. Omega-3 Rich Fatty Acids: Rich in chia seeds, flaxseeds, and fatty seafood like salmon, omega-3 fatty acids are vital partners in the battle against inflammation. Their anti-inflammatory qualities are essential for maintaining healthy cardiovascular systems as well as the best possible cognitive function.

2. Antioxidant-Rich and Colorful Vegetables: Boldly colored veggies like bell peppers, kale, and spinach are not only aesthetically pleasing but also nutrient-dense. Packed with vitamins, minerals, and antioxidants, these veggies help lower oxidative stress, which is a major cause of chronic inflammation.

3. Turmeric and Ginger: These two flavorful, warming spices are powerful anti-inflammatory agents in addition to being beautiful to look at. Turmeric's primary ingredient, curcumin, has been well-researched for its capacity to alter inflammatory pathways, making it an essential component of any anti-inflammatory kitchen.

4. Whole Grains: Packed with fiber and minerals, whole grains such as quinoa, brown rice, and oats give dishes a satisfying depth. Their complex carbs complement the diet's general anti-inflammatory objectives by supplying steady energy and helping to maintain a stable blood sugar level.

5. Extra Virgin Olive Oil: A cornerstone of the Anti-Anti-Inflammatory diet is substituting heart-healthy fats for saturated ones, and extra virgin olive oil is a great match. Packed with antioxidants and monounsaturated fats, it enhances the taste of food while also supporting heart health.

6. Lean Proteins: Including lean proteins helps prevent inflammatory responses while maintaining a balanced dietary profile. Examples of lean proteins are chicken, beans, and lentils. These protein sources provide the necessary amino acids for healthy muscles without any of the possible negative effects of processed or high-fat meats.

7. Berries and Citrus Fruits: Rich in vitamins and bursting with color, berries and citrus fruits like oranges and grapefruits provide a delightful taste. Rich in antioxidants, these fruits add to the body's defense against inflammation by helping to shield cells from harm caused by inflammation.

These key components essentially act as the taste ambassadors for the Anti-Anti-Inflammatory way of life. People who consume a wide variety of nutrient-dense foods provide delicious meals and establish the groundwork for long-term health and energy. These carefully selected and masterfully blended components serve as the catalysts for a life-changing transition towards a more colorful and anti-inflammatory lifestyle.

In the kitchen, the skill of producing delicious meals depends not only on the quality of the materials but also on the skillful use of instruments and equipment. A well-stocked kitchen is a blank canvas on which culinary creations are created, and a recipe's result may be greatly influenced by the instruments used.

Accuracy in Preparation: Knives, cutting boards, and measuring spoons are basic kitchen necessities. These are the instruments used by craftsmen, which enable accurate and effective ingredient preparation. While measuring tools provide precision in producing well-balanced tastes, high-quality knives guarantee clean cuts and improve culinary enjoyment overall.

Culinary Alchemy with Cookware: One of the most important aspects of kitchen basics is the choice of cookware. Baking sheets, pots, and pans serve as the furnace for culinary magic, turning uncooked components into delectable dishes. Cookware's composition and design help to distribute heat evenly, avoiding hot patches and guaranteeing consistent cooking outcomes.

Efficiency-Boosting Machinery: A variety of electrical equipment is often found in modern kitchens, and these appliances increase efficiency. These appliances simplify procedures and save significant time and effort. They range from stand mixers for easy mixing and kneading to blenders and food processors for quick ingredient processing.

Temperature Mastery with Thermometers: Expertise in cooking is characterized by exact temperature control. Instant-read and oven-safe thermometers enable chefs to achieve the ideal doneness in baked products, meats, and delicate dishes. Every ingredient in a dish is guaranteed to be cooked to perfection because of this meticulous attention to temperature.

Presentation Excellence: Presentation equipment goes beyond the kitchen and gives a gourmet masterpiece the final touch. Chefs may display their creative abilities by using molds, piping bags, and garnishing equipment, which turn a dish from a simple meal into a visual beauty.

Tools and equipment are essentially the unsung heroes of the culinary world; they improve the art and allow cooks of all skill levels to explore new flavors and techniques with accuracy, efficiency, and inventive flair. A well-chosen assortment of cooking utensils is not only a financial commitment, but also a necessary ally in the quest for culinary mastery.

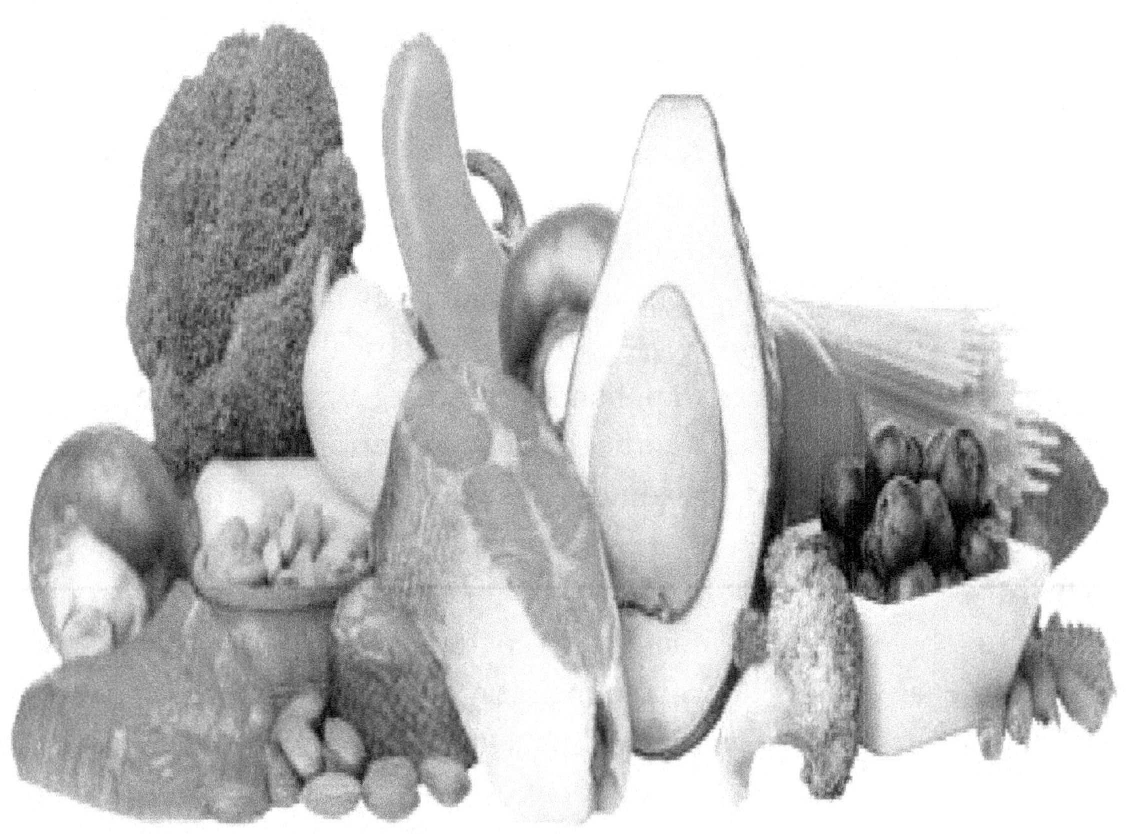

Chapter 3: Breakfast Delights

Berry Bliss Smoothie Bowl

INGREDIENTS

- ❖ 1 cup mixed berries (blueberries, strawberries, raspberries)
- ❖ 1 ripe banana
- ❖ 1/2 cup Greek yogurt
- ❖ 1 tablespoon chia seeds
- ❖ 1 teaspoon honey
- ❖ 1/2 cup almond milk

PREPARATION

- ❖ Blend berries, banana, Greek yogurt, chia seeds, and almond milk until smooth.
- ❖ Pour into a bowl and drizzle with honey.
- ❖ Top with additional berries and a sprinkle of chia seeds.

Nutrition Information

- ➢ Calories: 250
- ➢ Protein: 10g
- ➢ Fiber: 8g
- ➢ Antioxidants: High

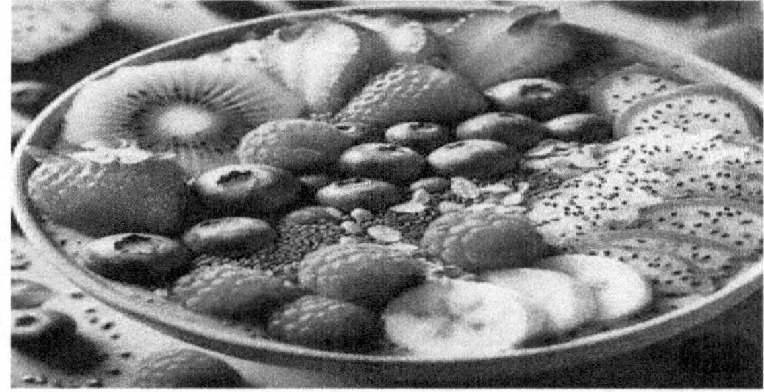

Turmeric Golden Oatmeal

INGREDIENTS

- ❖ 1 cup rolled oats
- ❖ 1/2 teaspoon turmeric powder
- ❖ 1/4 teaspoon cinnamon
- ❖ 1 tablespoon ground flaxseeds
- ❖ 1 tablespoon almond butter
- ❖ 1 cup almond milk

PREPARATION

- ❖ Cook oats with turmeric, cinnamon, and almond milk until creamy.
- ❖ Stir in flaxseeds and top with a dollop of almond butter.

Nutrition Information

- ➢ Calories: 280
- ➢ Protein: 9g
- ➢ Fiber: 7g
- ➢ Anti-Inflammatory Compounds: Turmeric

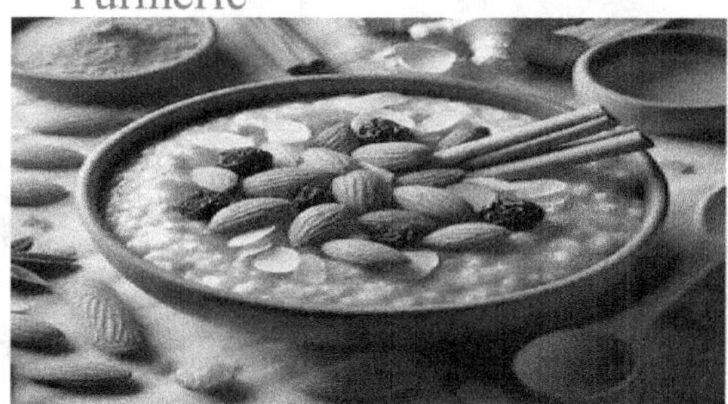

Avocado Toast with Poached Egg

INGREDIENTS

- 1 slice whole-grain bread
- 1/2 ripe avocado, mashed
- 1 poached egg
- Sprinkle of red pepper flakes
- Salt and pepper to taste

PREPARATION

- Toast the bread and spread mashed avocado.
- Top with a poached egg and season with red pepper flakes, salt, and pepper.

Nutrition Information

- Calories: 220
- Protein: 10g
- Healthy Fats: Avocado

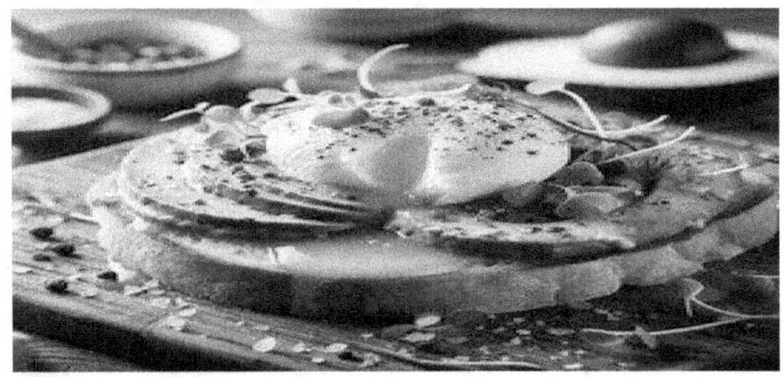

Chia Seed Pudding with Almond Butter

INGREDIENTS

- 3 tablespoons chia seeds
- 1 cup unsweetened coconut milk
- 1/2 teaspoon vanilla extract
- 1 tablespoon almond butter
- Fresh berries for topping

PREPARATION

- Mix chia seeds, coconut milk, and vanilla extract. Let it sit in the fridge for a few hours or overnight.
- Stir in almond butter before serving and top with fresh berries.

Nutrition Information

- Calories: 220
- Protein: 6g
- Omega-3 Fatty Acids: Chia Seeds

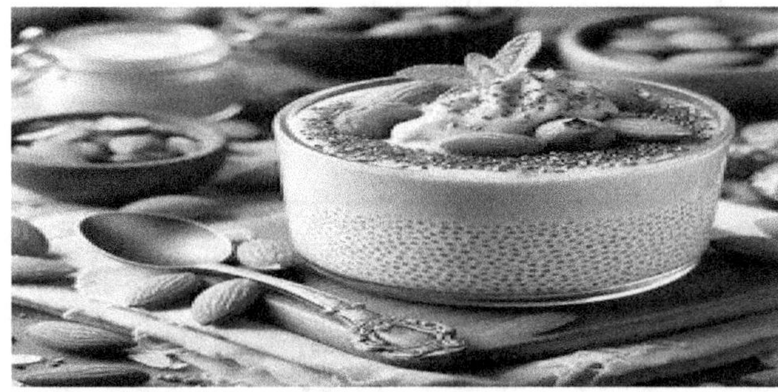

Quinoa Breakfast Bowl

INGREDIENTS

- ❖ 1/2 cup cooked quinoa
- ❖ 1/4 cup sliced almonds
- ❖ 1/2 cup mixed berries
- ❖ 1 tablespoon honey
- ❖ 1/2 cup Greek yogurt

PREPARATION

- ❖ Combine quinoa, almonds, and berries in a bowl.
- ❖ Drizzle with honey and top with a dollop of Greek yogurt.

Nutrition Information

- ➢ Calories: 280
- ➢ Protein: 12g
- ➢ Fiber: 5g
- ➢ Antioxidants: High

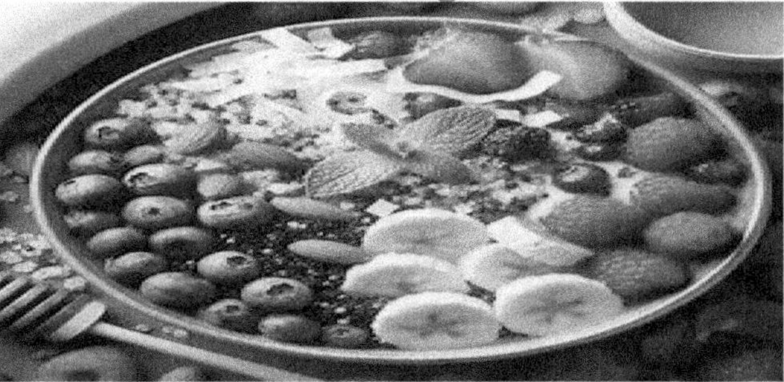

Spinach and Tomato Breakfast Wrap

INGREDIENTS

- ❖ 1 whole-grain wrap
- ❖ 2 large eggs, scrambled
- ❖ Handful of fresh spinach
- ❖ Sliced cherry tomatoes
- ❖ 1/4 cup feta cheese
- ❖ Salt and pepper to taste

PREPARATION

- ❖ Sauté spinach until wilted and set aside.
- ❖ Scramble eggs and assemble the wrap with eggs, spinach, tomatoes, and feta.
- ❖ Season with salt and pepper to taste.

Nutrition Information

- ➢ Calories: 320
- ➢ Protein: 18g
- ➢ Calcium: 15% DV

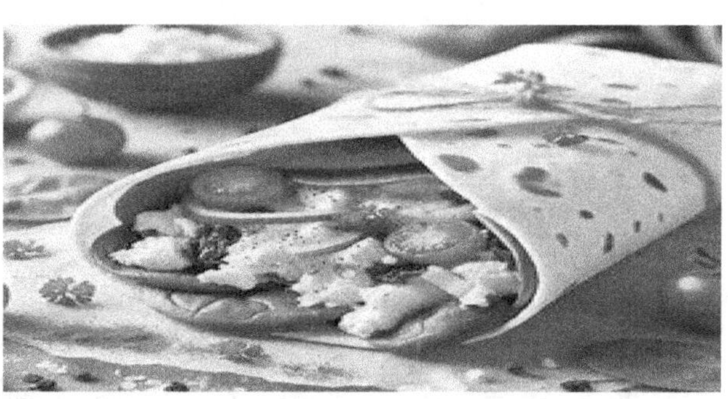

Coconut-Berry Chia Parfait

INGREDIENTS

- ❖ 1/2 cup coconut milk
- ❖ 2 tablespoons chia seeds
- ❖ 1/4 cup granola
- ❖ Mixed berries for layering
- ❖ 1 tablespoon shredded coconut

PREPARATION

- ❖ Mix chia seeds with coconut milk and let it set in the fridge.
- ❖ In a glass, layer chia pudding, granola, and mixed berries.
- ❖ Top with shredded coconut before serving.

Nutrition Information

- ➤ Calories: 280
- ➤ Protein: 6g
- ➤ Dietary Fiber: 8g

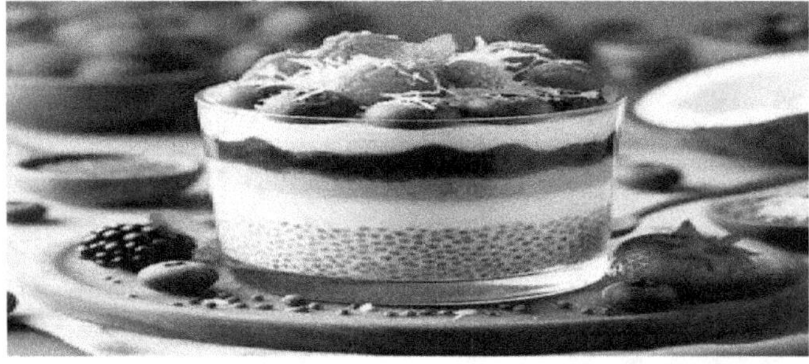

Sweet Potato and Kale Breakfast Hash

INGREDIENTS

- ❖ 1 medium sweet potato, diced
- ❖ 1 cup kale, chopped
- ❖ 1/2 red onion, diced
- ❖ 2 eggs
- ❖ 1 tablespoon olive oil
- ❖ Salt and pepper to taste

PREPARATION

- ❖ Sauté sweet potatoes and onions in olive oil until tender.
- ❖ Add kale and cook until wilted.
- ❖ Create wells in the hash, crack eggs into them, and cook until desired doneness.

Nutrition Information

- ➤ Calories: 310
- ➤ Protein: 10g
- ➤ Vitamin A: 150% DV

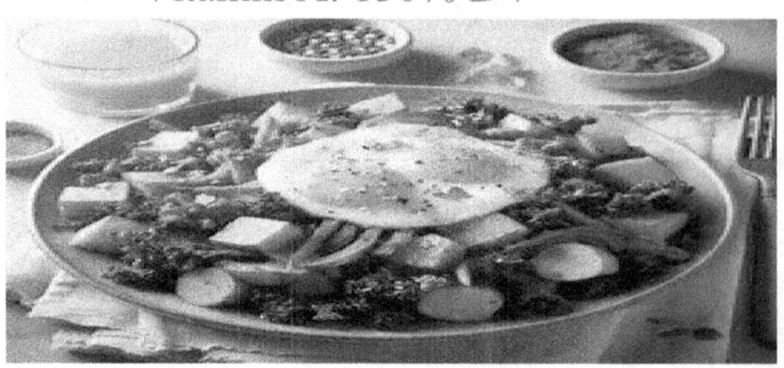

Cinnamon Apple Quinoa Bowl

INGREDIENTS

- ❖ 1/2 cup cooked quinoa
- ❖ 1 apple, diced
- ❖ 1 tablespoon almond butter
- ❖ Sprinkle of cinnamon
- ❖ 1/4 cup chopped walnuts

PREPARATION

- ❖ Combine quinoa, diced apple, and almond butter in a bowl.
- ❖ Sprinkle with cinnamon and top with chopped walnuts.

Nutrition Information

- ➢ Calories: 280
- ➢ Protein: 8g
- ➢ Healthy Fats: Almond Butter

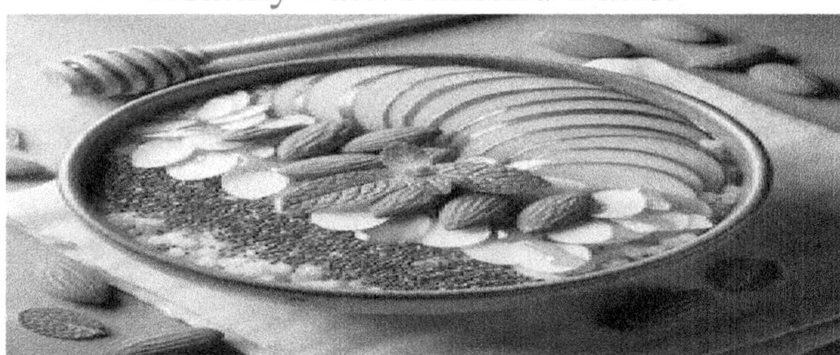

Mango Turmeric Overnight Oats

INGREDIENTS

- ❖ 1/2 cup rolled oats
- ❖ 1/2 cup diced mango
- ❖ 1/2 teaspoon turmeric powder
- ❖ 1 tablespoon honey
- ❖ 1/2 cup coconut milk

PREPARATION

- ❖ Mix oats, mango, turmeric, honey, and coconut milk in a jar.
- ❖ Refrigerate overnight and enjoy in the morning.

Nutrition Information

- ➢ Calories: 250
- ➢ Protein: 6g
- ➢ Vitamin C: 30% DV

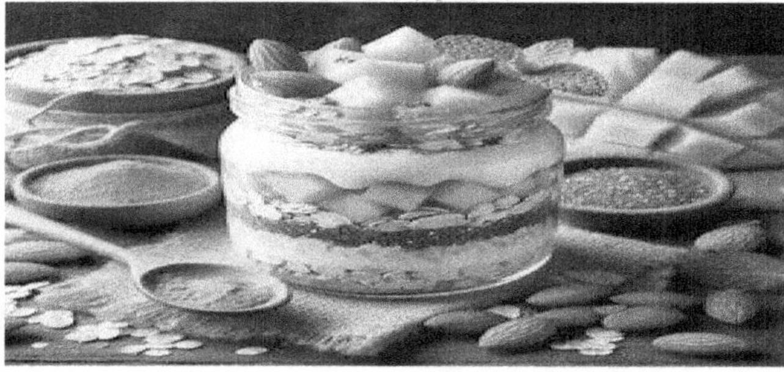

Chapter 4: Lunchtime Favorites

Grilled Salmon Salad Bowl

INGREDIENTS

- ❖ 1 cup mixed greens
- ❖ 6 oz grilled salmon fillet
- ❖ 1/2 cup cherry tomatoes, halved
- ❖ 1/4 cup cucumber, sliced
- ❖ 1/4 cup red bell pepper, diced
- ❖ 1 tablespoon extra-virgin olive oil
- ❖ 1 tablespoon balsamic vinegar
- ❖ Salt and pepper to taste

PREPARATION

- ❖ In a bowl, toss mixed greens, cherry tomatoes, cucumber, and red bell pepper.
- ❖ Top with grilled salmon.
- ❖ In a small bowl, whisk together olive oil, balsamic vinegar, salt, and pepper.
- ❖ Drizzle dressing over the salad and toss gently.
- ❖ Serve immediately.

Nutrition Information

- ➢ Calories: 350
- ➢ Protein: 30g
- ➢ Fat: 20g
- ➢ Carbohydrates: 15g
- ➢ Fiber: 5g

Quinoa and Chickpea Buddha Bowl

INGREDIENTS

- ❖ 1 cup cooked quinoa
- ❖ 1/2 cup chickpeas, roasted
- ❖ 1/2 cup kale, massaged
- ❖ 1/4 cup carrots, shredded
- ❖ 1/4 cup avocado, sliced
- ❖ 2 tablespoons tahini dressing
- ❖ Lemon juice for drizzling
- ❖ Salt and pepper to taste

PREPARATION

- ❖ Arrange quinoa, chickpeas, kale, carrots, and avocado in a bowl.
- ❖ Drizzle with tahini dressing and lemon juice.
- ❖ Season with salt and pepper.
- ❖ Toss gently before serving.

Nutrition Information

- ➢ Calories: 420
- ➢ Protein: 15g
- ➢ Fat: 18g
- ➢ Carbohydrates: 55g
- ➢ Fiber: 10g

Turmeric Chicken Wrap

INGREDIENTS

- ❖ 4 oz grilled chicken breast, sliced
- ❖ 1 whole-grain wrap
- ❖ 1/4 cup hummus
- ❖ 1/4 cup spinach
- ❖ 1/4 cup red cabbage, shredded
- ❖ 1/4 cup cucumber, julienned
- ❖ 1 teaspoon turmeric powder
- ❖ Salt and pepper to taste

PREPARATION

- ❖ Spread hummus on the wrap.
- ❖ Layer with spinach, grilled chicken, red cabbage, and cucumber.
- ❖ Sprinkle turmeric powder, salt, and pepper.
- ❖ Wrap tightly and cut in half.

Nutrition Information

- ➢ Calories: 380
- ➢ Protein: 30g
- ➢ Fat: 12g
- ➢ Carbohydrates: 40g
- ➢ Fiber: 8g

Mango Avocado Quinoa Salad

INGREDIENTS

- ❖ 1 cup cooked quinoa
- ❖ 1/2 ripe mango, diced
- ❖ 1/2 avocado, cubed
- ❖ 1/4 cup red onion, finely chopped
- ❖ 1/4 cup fresh cilantro, chopped
- ❖ 2 tablespoons lime juice
- ❖ 1 tablespoon extra-virgin olive oil
- ❖ Salt and pepper to taste

PREPARATION

- ❖ In a large bowl, combine quinoa, mango, avocado, red onion, and cilantro.
- ❖ In a small bowl, whisk together lime juice, olive oil, salt, and pepper.
- ❖ Pour the dressing over the salad and toss gently.
- ❖ Chill before serving for enhanced flavors.

Nutrition Information

- ➢ Calories: 320
- ➢ Protein: 8g
- ➢ Fat: 15g
- ➢ Carbohydrates: 40g
- ➢ Fiber: 6g

Lentil and Vegetable Soup

INGREDIENTS

- ❖ 1 cup green lentils, cooked
- ❖ 1/2 cup carrots, diced
- ❖ 1/2 cup celery, chopped
- ❖ 1/2 cup zucchini, sliced
- ❖ 1/4 cup onion, finely chopped
- ❖ 2 cloves garlic, minced
- ❖ 4 cups vegetable broth
- ❖ 1 teaspoon turmeric
- ❖ 1 teaspoon cumin
- ❖ Salt and pepper to taste

PREPARATION

- ❖ In a pot, sauté onions and garlic until fragrant.
- ❖ Add carrots, celery, and zucchini. Cook until vegetables soften.
- ❖ Stir in cooked lentils, vegetable broth, turmeric, cumin, salt, and pepper.
- ❖ Simmer for 20 minutes until flavors meld.

Nutrition Information

- ➢ Calories: 280
- ➢ Protein: 18g
- ➢ Fat: 2g
- ➢ Carbohydrates: 50g
- ➢ Fiber: 12g

Salmon and Asparagus Stir-Fry

INGREDIENTS

- ❖ 6 oz salmon fillet, cubed
- ❖ 1 cup asparagus, trimmed and cut into pieces
- ❖ 1/2 cup bell peppers, sliced
- ❖ 1/4 cup soy sauce (low-sodium)
- ❖ 1 tablespoon sesame oil
- ❖ 1 tablespoon ginger, minced
- ❖ 2 cloves garlic, minced
- ❖ 1 teaspoon honey
- ❖ Brown rice for serving

PREPARATION

- ❖ In a wok, heat sesame oil. Add ginger and garlic.
- ❖ Add salmon and stir-fry until cooked.
- ❖ Add asparagus and bell peppers. Cook until vegetables are tender-crisp.
- ❖ In a small bowl, mix soy sauce and honey. Pour over the stir-fry.
- ❖ Serve over brown rice.

Nutrition Information

- ➢ Calories: 380
- ➢ Protein: 28g
- ➢ Fat: 18g
- ➢ Carbohydrates: 25g
- ➢ Fiber: 5g

Chickpea and Spinach Curry

INGREDIENTS

- 1 can chickpeas, drained and rinsed
- 2 cups fresh spinach
- 1 onion, finely chopped
- 2 tomatoes, diced
- 1/4 cup coconut milk
- 2 tablespoons curry powder
- 1 tablespoon olive oil
- 1 teaspoon turmeric
- Salt and pepper to taste
- Basmati rice for serving

PREPARATION

- In a pan, sauté onions in olive oil until translucent.
- Add chickpeas, tomatoes, curry powder, turmeric, salt, and pepper. Cook for 5 minutes.
- Stir in spinach and coconut milk. Simmer until spinach wilts.
- Serve over basmati rice.

Nutrition Information

- Calories: 340
- Protein: 15g
- Fat: 10g
- Carbohydrates: 50g
- Fiber: 12g

Turkey and Sweet Potato Skillet

INGREDIENTS

- 1 lb ground turkey
- 2 sweet potatoes, diced
- 1 bell pepper, chopped
- 1 zucchini, sliced
- 1 tablespoon olive oil
- 1 teaspoon paprika
- 1 teaspoon rosemary
- Salt and pepper to taste

PREPARATION

- In a skillet, brown ground turkey in olive oil.
- Add sweet potatoes, bell pepper, zucchini, paprika, rosemary, salt, and pepper.
- Cook until sweet potatoes are tender and turkey is fully cooked.
- Serve hot.

Nutrition Information

- Calories: 320
- Protein: 25g
- Fat: 12g
- Carbohydrates: 30g
- Fiber: 6g

Mushroom and Spinach Stuffed Bell Peppers

INGREDIENTS

- ❖ 4 bell peppers, halved
- ❖ 1 cup mushrooms, chopped
- ❖ 2 cups fresh spinach, chopped
- ❖ 1 cup quinoa, cooked
- ❖ 1/4 cup feta cheese, crumbled
- ❖ 2 tablespoons olive oil
- ❖ 1 teaspoon Italian seasoning
- ❖ Salt and pepper to taste

PREPARATION

- ❖ Preheat oven to 375°F (190°C).
- ❖ In a pan, sauté mushrooms and spinach in olive oil.
- ❖ In a bowl, mix cooked quinoa, sautéed vegetables, feta, Italian seasoning, salt, and pepper.
- ❖ Stuff bell peppers with the mixture.
- ❖ Bake for 25-30 minutes until peppers are tender.

Nutrition Information

- ➢ Calories: 280
- ➢ Protein: 10g
- ➢ Fat: 12g
- ➢ Carbohydrates: 35g
- ➢ Fiber: 6g

Cauliflower and Chickpea Curry Bowl

INGREDIENTS

- ❖ 1 cup cauliflower florets
- ❖ 1 can chickpeas, drained and rinsed
- ❖ 1 cup cherry tomatoes, halved
- ❖ 1/2 cup coconut milk
- ❖ 1 tablespoon curry powder
- ❖ 1 tablespoon olive oil
- ❖ 2 cloves garlic, minced
- ❖ 1 teaspoon ginger, minced
- ❖ Basmati rice for serving

PREPARATION

- ❖ In a pan, sauté garlic and ginger in olive oil.
- ❖ Add cauliflower, chickpeas, cherry tomatoes, curry powder, and coconut milk. Simmer until cauliflower is tender.
- ❖ Serve over basmati rice.

Nutrition Information

- ➢ Calories: 330
- ➢ Protein: 15g
- ➢ Fat: 12g
- ➢ Carbohydrates: 45g
- ➢ Fiber: 10g

Chapter 5: Family-Friendly Dinners

Grilled Salmon with Turmeric Quinoa

INGREDIENTS

- ❖ 4 salmon fillets
- ❖ 1 cup quinoa
- ❖ 2 cups vegetable broth
- ❖ 1 tablespoon turmeric
- ❖ 1 tablespoon olive oil
- ❖ Salt and pepper to taste
- ❖ Lemon wedges for serving

PREPARATION

- ❖ Rinse quinoa under cold water and cook in vegetable broth with turmeric.
- ❖ Season salmon with salt, pepper, and olive oil. Grill until cooked through.
- ❖ Serve grilled salmon over turmeric quinoa.
- ❖ Garnish with fresh lemon wedges.

Nutrition Information

- ➢ Calories: 400
- ➢ Protein: 35g
- ➢ Carbohydrates: 30g
- ➢ Fiber: 4g
- ➢ Fat: 16g

Mushroom and Spinach Stuffed Chicken Breast

INGREDIENTS

- ❖ 4 chicken breasts
- ❖ 2 cups spinach, chopped
- ❖ 1 cup mushrooms, diced
- ❖ 2 cloves garlic, minced
- ❖ 1 tablespoon olive oil
- ❖ 1 teaspoon rosemary
- ❖ Salt and pepper to taste

PREPARATION

- ❖ Preheat oven to 375°F (190°C).
- ❖ In a pan, sauté garlic, spinach, and mushrooms in olive oil until wilted.
- ❖ Cut a pocket into each chicken breast and stuff with sautéed mixture.
- ❖ Season with rosemary, salt, and pepper.
- ❖ Bake until chicken is cooked through.

Nutrition Information

- ➢ Calories: 320
- ➢ Protein: 40g
- ➢ Carbohydrates: 5g
- ➢ Fiber: 2g
- ➢ Fat: 15g

Vegetarian Lentil and Sweet Potato Stew

INGREDIENTS

- ❖ 1 cup dry green lentils
- ❖ 2 sweet potatoes, diced
- ❖ 1 onion, chopped
- ❖ 3 carrots, sliced
- ❖ 3 cloves garlic, minced
- ❖ 4 cups vegetable broth
- ❖ 1 teaspoon cumin
- ❖ Salt and pepper to taste

PREPARATION

- ❖ Combine lentils, sweet potatoes, onion, carrots, and garlic in a pot.
- ❖ Add vegetable broth and bring to a simmer.
- ❖ Season with cumin, salt, and pepper.
- ❖ Cook until lentils and vegetables are tender.

Nutrition Information

- ➢ Calories: 280
- ➢ Protein: 14g
- ➢ Carbohydrates: 55g
- ➢ Fiber: 15g
- ➢ Fat: 1g

Tofu and Vegetable Stir-Fry

INGREDIENTS

- ❖ 1 block tofu, cubed
- ❖ 2 cups broccoli florets
- ❖ 1 bell pepper, sliced
- ❖ 1 carrot, julienned
- ❖ 3 tablespoons soy sauce
- ❖ 1 tablespoon sesame oil
- ❖ 1 teaspoon ginger, minced
- ❖ 2 cloves garlic, minced

PREPARATION

- ❖ Sauté tofu in sesame oil until golden.
- ❖ Add broccoli, bell pepper, ginger, and garlic. Stir-fry until vegetables are tender.
- ❖ Stir in soy sauce and cook for an additional 2 minutes.
- ❖ Serve over brown rice or quinoa.

Nutrition Information

- ➢ Calories: 320
- ➢ Protein: 20g
- ➢ Carbohydrates: 25g
- ➢ Fiber: 8g
- ➢ Fat: 18g

Chickpea and Spinach Curry

INGREDIENTS

- ❖ 2 cans chickpeas, drained
- ❖ 3 cups spinach
- ❖ 1 onion, chopped
- ❖ 2 tomatoes, diced
- ❖ 3 tablespoons curry powder
- ❖ 1 teaspoon turmeric
- ❖ 1 can coconut milk
- ❖ Salt and pepper to taste

PREPARATION

- ❖ Sauté onion in a pan until translucent.
- ❖ Add chickpeas, spinach, tomatoes, curry powder, and turmeric. Cook until spinach wilts.
- ❖ Stir in coconut milk and simmer until flavors meld.
- ❖ Season with salt and pepper.

Nutrition Information

- ➢ Calories: 380
- ➢ Protein: 15g
- ➢ Carbohydrates: 45g
- ➢ Fiber: 12g
- ➢ Fat: 18g

Quinoa and Black Bean Stuffed Peppers

INGREDIENTS

- ❖ 4 bell peppers, halved
- ❖ 1 cup quinoa, cooked
- ❖ 1 can black beans, drained
- ❖ 1 cup corn kernels
- ❖ 1 cup salsa
- ❖ 1 teaspoon cumin
- ❖ 1 teaspoon chili powder
- ❖ Shredded cheese (optional)

PREPARATION

- ❖ Preheat oven to 375°F (190°C).
- ❖ In a bowl, mix quinoa, black beans, corn, salsa, cumin, and chili powder.
- ❖ Stuff pepper halves with the mixture.
- ❖ Bake until peppers are tender. Top with cheese if desired.

Nutrition Information

- ➢ Calories: 290
- ➢ Protein: 12g
- ➢ Carbohydrates: 55g
- ➢ Fiber: 10g
- ➢ Fat: 3g

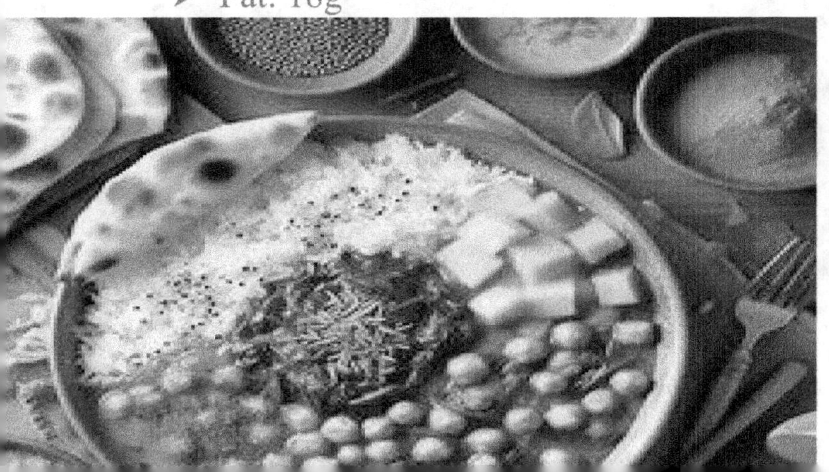
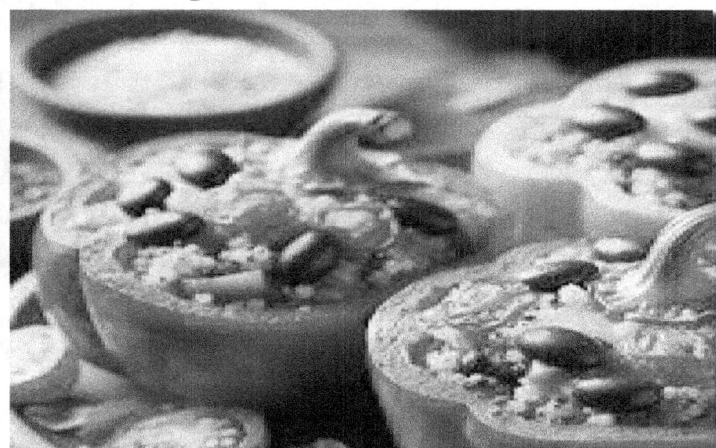

Salmon and Asparagus Foil Packets

INGREDIENTS

- ❖ 4 salmon fillets
- ❖ 1 bunch asparagus, trimmed
- ❖ 2 tablespoons olive oil
- ❖ 2 lemons, sliced
- ❖ 4 cloves garlic, minced
- ❖ Fresh dill for garnish
- ❖ Salt and pepper to taste

PREPARATION

- ❖ Preheat oven to 400°F (200°C).
- ❖ Place each salmon fillet on a piece of foil.
- ❖ Arrange asparagus around the salmon. Drizzle with olive oil.
- ❖ Season with minced garlic, salt, and pepper. Top with lemon slices.
- ❖ Seal the foil packets and bake until salmon is cooked.

Nutrition Information

- ➢ Calories: 350
- ➢ Protein: 30g
- ➢ Carbohydrates: 10g
- ➢ Fiber: 4g
- ➢ Fat: 20g

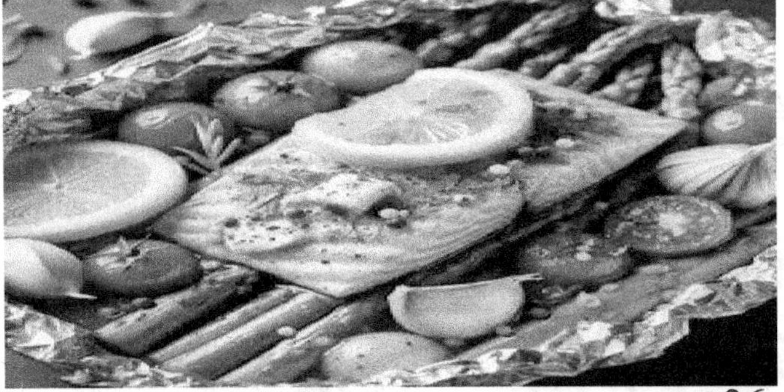

Vegetable and Chickpea Quinoa Bowl

INGREDIENTS

- ❖ 2 cups cooked quinoa
- ❖ 1 can chickpeas, drained
- ❖ 1 zucchini, diced
- ❖ 1 yellow squash, diced
- ❖ 1 cup cherry tomatoes, halved
- ❖ 1 cucumber, sliced
- ❖ Feta cheese for garnish
- ❖ Balsamic vinaigrette dressing

PREPARATION

- ❖ In a bowl, combine quinoa, chickpeas, zucchini, squash, tomatoes, and cucumber.
- ❖ Drizzle with balsamic vinaigrette and toss to combine.
- ❖ Garnish with feta cheese before serving.

Nutrition Information

- ➢ Calories: 320
- ➢ Protein: 14g
- ➢ Carbohydrates: 55g
- ➢ Fiber: 12g
- ➢ Fat: 8g

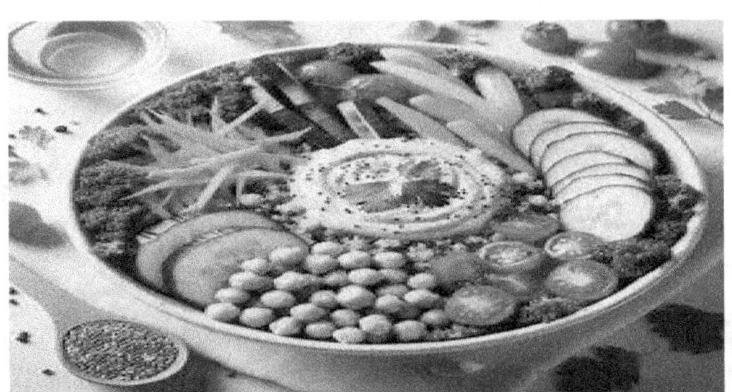

Lemon Garlic Shrimp with Whole Grain Pasta

INGREDIENTS

- ❖ 1 pound shrimp, peeled and deveined
- ❖ 2 cups whole grain pasta, cooked
- ❖ 3 tablespoons olive oil
- ❖ 4 cloves garlic, minced
- ❖ Zest and juice of 1 lemon
- ❖ Red pepper flakes (optional)
- ❖ Fresh parsley for garnish
- ❖ Salt and pepper to taste

PREPARATION

- ❖ Cook pasta according to package instructions.
- ❖ In a pan, sauté shrimp in olive oil with minced garlic until pink.
- ❖ Toss cooked pasta with shrimp, lemon zest, lemon juice, and red pepper flakes.
- ❖ Season with salt and pepper. Garnish with fresh parsley.

Nutrition Information

- ➢ Calories: 400
- ➢ Protein: 25g
- ➢ Carbohydrates: 45g
- ➢ Fiber: 8g
- ➢ Fat: 15g

Eggplant and Chickpea Curry

INGREDIENTS

- ❖ 1 large eggplant, diced
- ❖ 1 can chickpeas, drained
- ❖ 1 onion, chopped
- ❖ 2 tomatoes, diced
- ❖ 1 can coconut milk
- ❖ 3 tablespoons curry powder
- ❖ 1 teaspoon cumin
- ❖ Fresh cilantro for garnish
- ❖ Salt and pepper to taste

PREPARATION

- ❖ Sauté onion in a pan until softened.
- ❖ Add eggplant, chickpeas, tomatoes, curry powder, and cumin. Cook until eggplant is tender.
- ❖ Pour in coconut milk and simmer until flavors meld.
- ❖ Season with salt and pepper. Garnish with fresh cilantro.

Nutrition Information

- ➢ Calories: 350
- ➢ Protein: 10g
- ➢ Carbohydrates: 45g
- ➢ Fiber: 15g
- ➢ Fat: 18g

Chapter 6: Snack Attack

Turmeric-Spiced Roasted Chickpeas

INGREDIENTS

- ❖ 1 can (15 oz) chickpeas, drained and rinsed
- ❖ 1 tablespoon olive oil
- ❖ 1 teaspoon ground turmeric
- ❖ 1/2 teaspoon smoked paprika
- ❖ Salt and pepper to taste

PREPARATION

- ❖ Preheat the oven to 400°F (200°C).
- ❖ Pat dry the chickpeas with a paper towel to remove excess moisture.
- ❖ In a bowl, toss chickpeas with olive oil, turmeric, smoked paprika, salt, and pepper until evenly coated.
- ❖ Spread the chickpeas on a baking sheet in a single layer.
- ❖ Roast for 25-30 minutes or until golden and crispy, stirring halfway through.

Nutrition Information

- ➢ Calories: 120
- ➢ Protein: 5g
- ➢ Fiber: 4g
- ➢ Healthy Fats: 4g

Kale Chips with Garlic and Lemon

INGREDIENTS

- ❖ 1 bunch kale, stems removed and torn into bite-sized pieces
- ❖ 1 tablespoon olive oil
- ❖ 2 cloves garlic, minced
- ❖ Zest of 1 lemon
- ❖ Sea salt to taste

PREPARATION

- ❖ Preheat the oven to 350°F (175°C).
- ❖ In a large bowl, massage kale with olive oil, garlic, and lemon zest until well-coated.
- ❖ Spread kale on a baking sheet in a single layer.
- ❖ Bake for 10-15 minutes or until crispy, checking to prevent burning.
- ❖ Sprinkle with sea salt before serving.

Nutrition Information

- ➢ Calories: 60
- ➢ Protein: 3g
- ➢ Fiber: 2g
- ➢ Vitamin C: 30% DV

Avocado and Tomato Salsa with Whole Grain Crackers

INGREDIENTS

- ❖ 2 ripe avocados, diced
- ❖ 1 cup cherry tomatoes, halved
- ❖ 1/4 cup red onion, finely chopped
- ❖ 1/4 cup fresh cilantro, chopped
- ❖ Juice of 1 lime
- ❖ Whole grain crackers for serving

PREPARATION

- ❖ In a bowl, combine diced avocados, cherry tomatoes, red onion, cilantro, and lime juice.
- ❖ Mix gently until well combined.
- ❖ Serve with whole grain crackers.

Nutrition Information

- ➢ Calories: 160
- ➢ Protein: 2g
- ➢ Healthy Fats: 12g
- ➢ Fiber: 6g

Greek Yogurt Parfait with Berries and Almonds

INGREDIENTS

- ❖ 1 cup Greek yogurt
- ❖ 1/2 cup mixed berries (blueberries, strawberries, raspberries)
- ❖ 2 tablespoons almonds, chopped
- ❖ 1 tablespoon honey

PREPARATION

- ❖ In a glass or bowl, layer Greek yogurt with mixed berries.
- ❖ Top with chopped almonds and drizzle with honey.

Nutrition Information

- ➢ Calories: 220
- ➢ Protein: 15g
- ➢ Healthy Fats: 10g
- ➢ Fiber: 4g

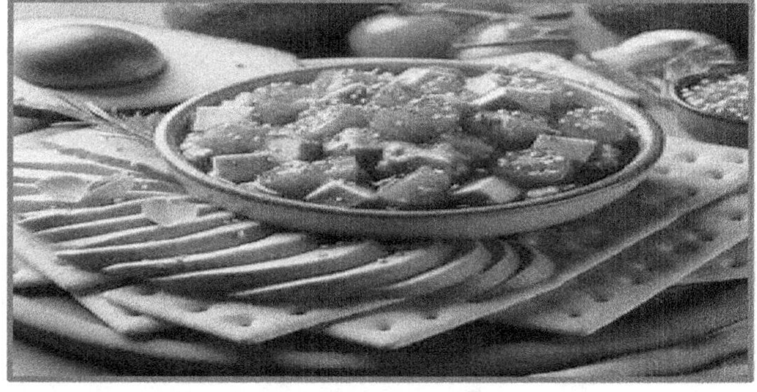

Cucumber and Hummus Bites

INGREDIENTS

- ❖ 1 cucumber, sliced
- ❖ 1/2 cup hummus
- ❖ Cherry tomatoes for garnish
- ❖ Fresh parsley, chopped

PREPARATION

- ❖ Arrange cucumber slices on a serving platter.
- ❖ Spoon a dollop of hummus onto each cucumber slice.
- ❖ Garnish with cherry tomatoes and chopped parsley.

Nutrition Information

- ➢ Calories: 70
- ➢ Protein: 3g
- ➢ Healthy Fats: 4g
- ➢ Fiber: 2g

Quinoa and Veggie Stuffed Bell Peppers

INGREDIENTS

- ❖ 3 bell peppers, halved and seeds removed
- ❖ 1 cup cooked quinoa
- ❖ 1/2 cup black beans, drained and rinsed
- ❖ 1/2 cup corn kernels
- ❖ 1/4 cup red onion, finely chopped
- ❖ 1/2 teaspoon cumin
- ❖ 1/2 teaspoon chili powder
- ❖ Salsa for topping

PREPARATION

- ❖ Preheat the oven to 375°F (190°C).
- ❖ In a bowl, mix cooked quinoa, black beans, corn, red onion, cumin, and chili powder.
- ❖ Stuff each bell pepper half with the quinoa mixture.
- ❖ Bake for 20-25 minutes or until peppers are tender.
- ❖ Top with salsa before serving.

Nutrition Information

- ➢ Calories: 180
- ➢ Protein: 7g
- ➢ Fiber: 6g
- ➢ Vitamin A: 100% DV

Edamame and Sea Salt Snack Bowl

INGREDIENTS

- ❖ 2 cups edamame, steamed and cooled
- ❖ Sea salt to taste
- ❖ Lemon wedges for squeezing

PREPARATION

- ❖ Place steamed edamame in a bowl.
- ❖ Sprinkle with sea salt to taste.
- ❖ Serve with lemon wedges for squeezing.

Nutrition Information

- ➢ Calories: 160
- ➢ Protein: 17g
- ➢ Healthy Fats: 8g
- ➢ Fiber: 8g

Chia Seed Pudding with Mixed Berries

INGREDIENTS

- ❖ 3 tablespoons chia seeds
- ❖ 1 cup almond milk
- ❖ 1/2 teaspoon vanilla extract
- ❖ 1 tablespoon maple syrup
- ❖ Mixed berries for topping

PREPARATION

- ❖ In a bowl, mix chia seeds, almond milk, vanilla extract, and maple syrup.
- ❖ Refrigerate for at least 4 hours or overnight until a pudding-like consistency is achieved.
- ❖ Top with mixed berries before serving.

Nutrition Information

- ➢ Calories: 180
- ➢ Protein: 4g
- ➢ Healthy Fats: 8g
- ➢ Fiber: 12g

Sweet Potato and Rosemary Baked Fries

INGREDIENTS

- ❖ 2 sweet potatoes, cut into fries
- ❖ 1 tablespoon olive oil
- ❖ 1 teaspoon dried rosemary
- ❖ Salt and pepper to taste

PREPARATION

- ❖ Preheat the oven to 400°F (200°C).
- ❖ In a bowl, toss sweet potato fries with olive oil, dried rosemary, salt, and pepper.
- ❖ Spread the fries on a baking sheet in a single layer.
- ❖ Bake for 25-30 minutes or until golden and crispy, flipping halfway through.

Nutrition Information

- ➢ Calories: 150
- ➢ Protein: 2g
- ➢ Healthy Fats: 5g
- ➢ Fiber: 4g

Spinach and Artichoke Dip with Whole Wheat Pita

INGREDIENTS

- ❖ 1 cup frozen chopped spinach, thawed and drained
- ❖ 1 can (14 oz) artichoke hearts, drained and chopped
- ❖ 1 cup Greek yogurt
- ❖ 1/2 cup grated Parmesan cheese
- ❖ 1/2 cup mozzarella cheese
- ❖ 1 clove garlic, minced
- ❖ Whole wheat pita for dipping

PREPARATION

- ❖ Preheat the oven to 375°F (190°C).
- ❖ In a bowl, mix spinach, artichoke hearts, Greek yogurt, Parmesan, mozzarella, and minced garlic.
- ❖ Transfer the mixture to a baking dish.
- ❖ Bake for 25-30 minutes or until bubbly and golden.
- ❖ Serve with whole wheat pita for dipping.

Nutrition Information

- ➢ Calories: 200
- ➢ Protein: 15g
- ➢ Healthy Fats: 8g
- ➢ Fiber: 5g

Chapter 7: Sweet Endings

Turmeric-infused Mango Sorbet

INGREDIENTS

- ❖ 2 ripe mangoes, peeled and diced
- ❖ 1 teaspoon turmeric powder
- ❖ 1/4 cup honey
- ❖ 1 cup coconut water

PREPARATION

- ❖ Blend mangoes, turmeric, honey, and coconut water until smooth.
- ❖ Pour the mixture into an ice cream maker and churn according to the manufacturer's instructions.
- ❖ Transfer to a container and freeze until firm.
- ❖ Scoop and serve for a delightful anti-inflammatory treat.

Nutrition Information

- ➢ Calories: 120
- ➢ Protein: 1g
- ➢ Fat: 0.5g
- ➢ Carbohydrates: 30g
- ➢ Fiber: 3g

Berry-licious Chia Pudding

INGREDIENTS

- ❖ 1/4 cup chia seeds
- ❖ 1 cup almond milk
- ❖ 1 cup mixed berries (blueberries, raspberries, strawberries)
- ❖ 1 tablespoon honey
- ❖ 1/2 teaspoon vanilla extract

PREPARATION

- ❖ Mix chia seeds, almond milk, honey, and vanilla extract in a bowl.
- ❖ Refrigerate for at least 4 hours or overnight.
- ❖ Layer the chia pudding with mixed berries.
- ❖ Garnish with extra berries and serve.

Nutrition Information

- ➢ Calories: 180
- ➢ Protein: 4g
- ➢ Fat: 8g
- ➢ Carbohydrates: 25g
- ➢ Fiber: 10g

Avocado Chocolate Mousse

INGREDIENTS

- ❖ 2 ripe avocados
- ❖ 1/4 cup cocoa powder
- ❖ 1/4 cup maple syrup
- ❖ 1 teaspoon vanilla extract
- ❖ A pinch of sea salt

PREPARATION

- ❖ Blend avocados, cocoa powder, maple syrup, vanilla extract, and salt until creamy.
- ❖ Chill in the refrigerator for 2 hours.
- ❖ Spoon into serving glasses and enjoy this decadent, anti-inflammatory chocolate mousse.

Nutrition Information

- ➢ Calories: 200
- ➢ Protein: 3g
- ➢ Fat: 15g
- ➢ Carbohydrates: 18g
- ➢ Fiber: 7g

Golden Apple Cinnamon Bites

INGREDIENTS

- ❖ 2 apples, thinly sliced
- ❖ 1 tablespoon coconut oil, melted
- ❖ 1 teaspoon ground cinnamon
- ❖ 1 tablespoon maple syrup
- ❖ A sprinkle of turmeric powder

PREPARATION

- ❖ Preheat the oven to 350°F (175°C).
- ❖ Toss apple slices with melted coconut oil, cinnamon, and maple syrup.
- ❖ Arrange on a baking sheet and bake for 15-20 minutes until apples are golden.
- ❖ Dust with turmeric powder for an extra anti-inflammatory boost.

Nutrition Information

- ➢ Calories: 90
- ➢ Protein: 0.5g
- ➢ Fat: 4g
- ➢ Carbohydrates: 15g
- ➢ Fiber: 3g

Pineapple Mint Sorbet Popsicles

INGREDIENTS

- ❖ 2 cups fresh pineapple chunks
- ❖ 1/4 cup fresh mint leaves
- ❖ 1 tablespoon lime juice
- ❖ 2 tablespoons honey
- ❖ 1/2 cup coconut water

PREPARATION

- ❖ Blend pineapple, mint, lime juice, honey, and coconut water until smooth.
- ❖ Pour into popsicle molds and freeze until solid.
- ❖ Unmold and savor these refreshing, anti-inflammatory popsicles.

Nutrition Information

- ➢ Calories: 60
- ➢ Protein: 0.5g
- ➢ Fat: 0.5g
- ➢ Carbohydrates: 15g
- ➢ Fiber: 1.5g

Cinnamon-Baked Pears with Almond Crumble

INGREDIENTS

- ❖ 4 ripe pears, halved
- ❖ 1 teaspoon ground cinnamon
- ❖ 1/4 cup almond flour
- ❖ 2 tablespoons melted coconut oil
- ❖ 1 tablespoon maple syrup

PREPARATION

- ❖ Preheat the oven to 375°F (190°C).
- ❖ Place pear halves on a baking sheet, sprinkle with cinnamon.
- ❖ In a bowl, mix almond flour, melted coconut oil, and maple syrup to create crumble.
- ❖ Top each pear half with crumble and bake for 20-25 minutes until golden.

Nutrition Information

- ➢ Fat: 7g
- ➢ Carbohydrates: 15g
- ➢ Fiber: 4g

Mixed Berry Parfait with Greek Yogurt

INGREDIENTS

- ❖ 1 cup mixed berries (strawberries, blueberries, raspberries)
- ❖ 1 cup Greek yogurt
- ❖ 2 tablespoons honey
- ❖ 1/4 cup granola

PREPARATION

- ❖ In a glass, layer Greek yogurt, mixed berries, and drizzle with honey.
- ❖ Repeat the layers.
- ❖ Top with granola for added crunch and serve.

Nutrition Information

- ➢ Calories: 180
- ➢ Protein: 12g
- ➢ Fat: 5g
- ➢ Carbohydrates: 25g
- ➢ Fiber: 4g

Chocolate Avocado Truffles

INGREDIENTS

- ❖ 2 ripe avocados
- ❖ 1/4 cup unsweetened cocoa powder
- ❖ 2 tablespoons honey
- ❖ 1/2 teaspoon vanilla extract
- ❖ A pinch of sea salt
- ❖ Shredded coconut for coating (optional)

PREPARATION

- ❖ Mash avocados and mix with cocoa powder, honey, vanilla extract, and salt.
- ❖ Form into small truffles and roll in shredded coconut if desired.
- ❖ Chill in the refrigerator before serving.

Nutrition Information

- ➢ Calories: 120
- ➢ Protein: 2g
- ➢ Fat: 8g
- ➢ Carbohydrates: 15g
- ➢ Fiber: 5g

Anti-Inflammatory Peach Ginger Smoothie Bowl

INGREDIENTS

- ❖ 2 ripe peaches, sliced
- ❖ 1 frozen banana
- ❖ 1/2 cup Greek yogurt
- ❖ 1 teaspoon fresh ginger, grated
- ❖ 1 tablespoon chia seeds

PREPARATION

- ❖ Blend peaches, banana, Greek yogurt, and ginger until smooth.
- ❖ Pour into a bowl and top with chia seeds for added texture.

Nutrition Information

- ➢ Calories: 200
- ➢ Protein: 8g
- ➢ Fat: 5g
- ➢ Carbohydrates: 30g
- ➢ Fiber: 5g

Blueberry Almond Bliss Bars

INGREDIENTS

- ❖ 1 cup fresh or frozen blueberries
- ❖ 1 cup almonds, finely ground
- ❖ 1/4 cup coconut oil, melted
- ❖ 2 tablespoons honey
- ❖ 1 teaspoon vanilla extract

PREPARATION

- ❖ Blend blueberries, ground almonds, melted coconut oil, honey, and vanilla extract until a dough forms.
- ❖ Press the mixture into a lined baking dish and refrigerate until firm.
- ❖ Cut into bars and savor these antioxidant-rich delights.

Nutrition Information

- ➢ Calories: 150
- ➢ Protein: 4g
- ➢ Fat: 12g
- ➢ Carbohydrates: 10g

Grilled Turmeric Chicken Skewers

INGREDIENTS

- ❖ 1 pound boneless, skinless chicken breasts, cut into cubes
- ❖ 2 tablespoons olive oil
- ❖ 1 teaspoon ground turmeric
- ❖ 1 teaspoon ground cumin
- ❖ 1 teaspoon paprika
- ❖ Salt and pepper to taste
- ❖ Wooden skewers, soaked in water

PREPARATION

- ❖ In a bowl, mix olive oil, turmeric, cumin, paprika, salt, and pepper to create a marinade.
- ❖ Coat chicken cubes with the marinade and refrigerate for at least 30 minutes.
- ❖ Thread marinated chicken onto skewers.
- ❖ Grill skewers until chicken is cooked through, about 10 minutes, turning occasionally.

Nutrition Information

- ➢ Calories: 250
- ➢ Protein: 30g
- ➢ Carbohydrates: 2g
- ➢ Fat: 13g

Salmon with Lemon and Dill

INGREDIENTS

- ❖ 4 salmon fillets
- ❖ 2 tablespoons olive oil
- ❖ 1 tablespoon fresh dill, chopped
- ❖ Juice of 1 lemon
- ❖ Salt and pepper to taste

PREPARATION

- ❖ Preheat oven to 375°F (190°C).
- ❖ Place salmon fillets on a baking sheet.
- ❖ Drizzle olive oil and lemon juice over the salmon.
- ❖ Sprinkle with chopped dill, salt, and pepper.
- ❖ Bake for 15-20 minutes or until salmon flakes easily with a fork.

Nutrition Information

- ➢ Calories: 300
- ➢ Protein: 25g
- ➢ Carbohydrates: 1g
- ➢ Fat: 20g

Herb-Marinated Turkey Breast

INGREDIENTS

- 1.5 pounds turkey breast
- 3 tablespoons olive oil
- 1 tablespoon fresh thyme, chopped
- 1 tablespoon fresh sage, chopped
- 1 tablespoon fresh rosemary, chopped
- Salt and pepper to taste

PREPARATION

- Preheat the oven to 350°F (175°C).
- In a bowl, mix olive oil, thyme, sage, rosemary, salt, and pepper.
- Rub the mixture onto the turkey breast and bake for 1 hour or until the internal temperature reaches 165°F (74°C).

Nutrition Information

- Calories: 220
- Protein: 30g
- Carbohydrates: 0g
- Fat: 10g

Cumin-Spiced Beef Stir-Fry

INGREDIENTS

- 1 pound sirloin steak, thinly sliced
- 2 tablespoons soy sauce (low-sodium)
- 1 tablespoon ground cumin
- 1 tablespoon olive oil
- 1 bell pepper, sliced
- 1 cup broccoli florets

PREPARATION

- In a bowl, combine sliced steak with soy sauce and cumin. Marinate for 20 minutes.
- Heat olive oil in a wok or skillet over high heat.
- Stir-fry the marinated steak, bell pepper, and broccoli until cooked through.

Nutrition Information

- Calories: 290
- Protein: 30g
- Carbohydrates: 8g
- Fat: 14g

Lemon Garlic Shrimp Skewers

INGREDIENTS

- ❖ 1 pound large shrimp, peeled and deveined
- ❖ 3 tablespoons olive oil
- ❖ Zest and juice of 1 lemon
- ❖ 2 cloves garlic, minced
- ❖ Fresh parsley, chopped
- ❖ Salt and pepper to taste

PREPARATION

- ❖ In a bowl, mix olive oil, lemon zest, lemon juice, minced garlic, chopped parsley, salt, and pepper.
- ❖ Coat shrimp with the marinade and let it sit for 15-20 minutes.
- ❖ Thread marinated shrimp onto skewers and grill for 2-3 minutes per side.

Nutrition Information

- ➢ Calories: 180
- ➢ Protein: 22g
- ➢ Carbohydrates: 2g
- ➢ Fat: 9g

Balsamic Glazed Chicken Thighs

INGREDIENTS

- ❖ 1.5 pounds chicken thighs, bone-in, skin-on
- ❖ 1/4 cup balsamic vinegar
- ❖ 2 tablespoons honey
- ❖ 1 tablespoon olive oil
- ❖ 2 cloves garlic, minced
- ❖ 1 teaspoon dried thyme
- ❖ Salt and black pepper to taste

PREPARATION

- ❖ Preheat the oven to 400°F (200°C).
- ❖ In a bowl, whisk together balsamic vinegar, honey, olive oil, minced garlic, dried thyme, salt, and black pepper.
- ❖ Place chicken thighs in a baking dish, pour the balsamic mixture over them, and bake for 30-35 minutes.

Nutrition Information

- ➢ Calories: 280
- ➢ Protein: 25g
- ➢ Carbohydrates: 9g
- ➢ Fat: 16g

Mango Chili Lime Grilled Chicken

INGREDIENTS

- ❖ 1.5 pounds chicken breasts
- ❖ 1 ripe mango, peeled and mashed
- ❖ 2 tablespoons lime juice
- ❖ 1 tablespoon chili powder
- ❖ 1 teaspoon cayenne pepper (adjust to taste)
- ❖ Salt to taste

PREPARATION

- ❖ In a bowl, combine mashed mango, lime juice, chili powder, cayenne pepper, and salt.
- ❖ Coat chicken breasts with the marinade and refrigerate for at least 1 hour.
- ❖ Grill chicken until fully cooked, basting with the remaining marinade.

Nutrition Information

- ➢ Calories: 240
- ➢ Protein: 28g
- ➢ Carbohydrates: 15g
- ➢ Fat: 8g

Pesto Turkey Zucchini Boats

INGREDIENTS

- ❖ 1 pound ground turkey
- ❖ 4 medium zucchinis, halved
- ❖ 1/2 cup pesto sauce (homemade or store-bought)
- ❖ 1 cup cherry tomatoes, halved
- ❖ 1/2 cup feta cheese, crumbled
- ❖ Salt and pepper to taste

PREPARATION

- ❖ Preheat the oven to 375°F (190°C).
- ❖ Brown ground turkey in a skillet, season with salt and pepper.
- ❖ Scoop out the center of zucchini halves to create boats.
- ❖ Mix ground turkey with pesto, stuff into zucchini boats, and top with cherry tomatoes and feta.
- ❖ Bake for 20-25 minutes or until zucchini is tender.

Nutrition Information

- ➢ Calories: 320
- ➢ Protein: 28g
- ➢ Carbohydrates: 10g
- ➢ Fat: 18g

Chapter 9: Expert Endorsements

Pediatricians' perspectives provide an invaluable angle on how diet, health, and child development are intertwined. Pediatricians provide parents and other caregivers with vital advice because they are dependable advocates for the health of children. The following are some important observations made by physicians that provide light on building a sound foundation for kids:

1. Early Nutritional Influence: Early nutrition has a significant influence on a child's growth and development, as pediatricians stress. A child's early years are crucial for brain development, therefore it's important to feed them well at this time. Pediatricians' observations emphasize the requirement of nursing, starting solid foods at a young age, and eating balanced meals to suit a child's nutritional demands, which are essential for their general health.

2. Nutrient-Rich Diets for Growth: A range of food categories should be included in nutrient-rich diets, according to pediatricians. Protein, vitamins, minerals, and other essential nutrients are crucial for promoting healthy growth, cognitive development, and immune system performance. Parents may create well-balanced meals that meet the unique dietary needs of each developmental stage with the help of these medical professionals' insights.

3. Filling in Nutritional Gaps: Pediatricians locate and fill in any possible dietary gaps for children. Making sure you're getting enough micronutrients like iron, calcium, and vitamin D is part of this. Pediatricians' insights help parents choose a variety of meals to fill in nutritional deficiencies and, when needed, provide supplements that are suitable for a child's age and health.

4. Preventing Childhood Obesity: Child health professionals are essential in managing and preventing childhood obesity. They shed light on sensible eating practices, sensible portion sizes, and the value of consistent exercise. These realizations assist parents in establishing a setting that supports a healthy weight and lowers the likelihood of obesity-related health problems in children and adults.

5. Managing Food Allergies: Pediatricians' insights are very helpful in identifying and treating food allergies in kids. When necessary, they provide advice to parents on how to recognize allergies, appropriately introduce solid meals, and create settings free of allergens. Pediatricians collaborate closely with families to create individualized meal plans that provide the best possible nutrition and account for dietary restrictions.

6. Teaching Good Eating Habits: Pediatricians are also teachers, passing along important information about developing good eating habits at a young age. The medical specialists' insights recommend that a child's diet include a range of fruits, vegetables, whole grains, and lean meats. They emphasize how crucial it is to set a good example for healthy eating within the family to create enduring habits.

7. Monitoring Growth and Development: Recognizing that nutrition is a dynamic part of overall health, pediatricians regularly evaluate a child's growth and development. Personalized guidance may be given during routine examinations, guaranteeing that a child's dietary requirements are satisfied from early childhood through puberty.

Parents might think of physicians' views as a kind of compass that helps them navigate the complex world of kid nutrition. By paying attention to these observations, caregivers may create an atmosphere that promotes optimum health, giving the youngest members of society the basis for a lifetime of well-being.

The "Anti-Anti-Inflammatory Cookbook" is a carefully composed symphony of tastes based on scientific accuracy, not merely a compilation of delicious dishes. Inspired by the most recent discoveries in health research, each dish in these pages is the product of a sophisticated grasp of the complex interactions between inflammation and nutrition.

The scientific method used in the cookbook's ingredient selection is its cornerstone. Each component is selected for its unique anti-inflammatory qualities in addition to its gastronomic appeal. The dishes, which range from omega-3 fatty acid-rich fish to antioxidant-rich berries, are a purposeful combination of nutrients intended to actively combat chronic inflammation in the body.

The meticulous macronutrient balance in the meals is another example of the science at work. With a thoughtful mix of healthy fats, proteins, and carbs, the cookbook promises to provide not just a satisfying meal but also one that is well-balanced. This equilibrium has been carefully chosen by scientists to promote long-term energy levels, preserve a healthy body composition, and enhance general well-being.

Knowing how carbs affect inflammation, the cookbook takes a careful approach to glycemic management. The recipes try to control blood sugar levels by using complex carbs that have a lower glycemic index. This reduces the risk of inflammation that comes with irregular blood sugar rises.

The recipes' science extends to the cooking area as well, with a focus on methods that optimize nutrient retention. Every technique, from selecting to steam instead of fry to adding uncooked ingredients for additional enzymatic advantages, is a deliberate choice based on scientific knowledge.

Known for their anti-inflammatory qualities, adaptogenic herbs and spices are a standout addition to the recipe. The use of these organic components is a tribute to the scientifically proven therapeutic power of nature, from ginger's strong anti-inflammatory properties to turmeric's curcumin concentration.

Essentially, the "Anti-Anti-Inflammatory Cookbook" is a celebration of the union of science and cuisine, not only a tour de cuisine. When the science of nutrition and the art of cooking are combined, every meal becomes a tasty prescription for health, enticing people to enjoy not only the flavor but also the many health advantages that are included in each culinary masterpiece.

Conclusion

Coming to the end of the "Anti-Anti-Inflammatory Cookbook for Family," we wrap up our culinary adventure full of hope and a strong sense of purpose. This book is a manifesto for the transforming potential of deliberate, health-conscious living, not just a compilation of recipes. Let's connect the dots between the expertly prepared meals and the scientific ideas that informed them as we consider the themes that ran throughout this culinary journey.

The Anti-Anti-Inflammatory approach's core ideas transcend conventional dietary paradigms. It captures a comprehensive view of health, recognizing the complex relationship between diet, inflammation, and general well-being. Adopting this strategy will cause a significant change in your family's perspective and experience of well-being, not just in what's on your plate.

This cookbook promotes the notion that fueling your body can be a celebration of taste and joy, dispelling the myth that eating healthfully equals gourmet hardship. Every dish demonstrates the harmonious combination of flavor and nutrition, demonstrating that pursuing well-being does not always require making sacrifices. The culinary scene shown here, which ranges from colorful breakfasts to lavish meals and mouthwatering sweets, is a canvas for the skillful fusion of health and cuisine.

The pediatrician's seal of approval highlights the dedication to family health that permeates every aspect of this cookbook. We guarantee that the recipes collected within these pages exceed the highest standards of nutritional quality and safety by harmonizing with the experience of medical specialists. The endorsement serves as more than simply confirmation; it is evidence of the commitment to each family member's well-being and health.

Think of this as a call to action as well as a conclusion when the last few pages unfold. The anti-inflammatory method is a sustainable way of living rather than a fad. The recipes that are offered are not strict guidelines; rather, they are calls to experiment, personalize, and integrate healthy options into your family's everyday routine. This cookbook serves as a guide, and you are the author of the continuous story of your path toward long-term well-being.

We encourage you to promote the Anti-Anti-Inflammatory approach's tenets for the sake of vibrant health, mindful eating, and the limitless possibilities for revolutionary transformation. In the future, when every meal is an opportunity for nutrition, every decision is a stride toward well-being, and your family's health becomes a legacy of purposeful, health-conscious living, may this book serve as a compass for you. Cheers to the Anti-Anti-Inflammatory journey's transforming power that permeates all aspects of your family's existence and transcends the kitchen.

Appendix

Measurement Conversions

Length:

- 1 inch = 2.54 centimeters
- 1 foot = 0.3048 meters
- 1 mile = 1.609 kilometers

Weight:

- 1 pound = 0.4536 kilograms
- 1 ounce = 28.35 grams
- 1 ton (US) = 907.185 kilograms

Volume (Liquid):

- 1 fluid ounce = 29.573 milliliters
- 1 cup = 240 milliliters
- 1 gallon = 3.785 liters

Volume (Dry):

- 1 teaspoon = 5.919 milliliters
- 1 tablespoon = 17.757 milliliters
- 1 quart = 1.101 liters

Temperature:

- Celsius to Fahrenheit: $°F = (°C × 9/5) + 32$
- Fahrenheit to Celsius: $°C = (°F - 32) × 5/9$

Time:

- 1 minute = 60 seconds
- 1 hour = 60 minutes
- 1 day = 24 hours

Speed:

- 1 mile per hour = 1.609 kilometers per hour
- 1 meter per second = 3.281 feet per second

1. Flour:
- **All-Purpose Flour:** Whole wheat flour, almond flour, coconut flour, or gluten-free flour blend.
- **Bread Flour:** All-purpose flour with a dash of vital wheat gluten for added protein.
- **Cake Flour:** A mixture of all-purpose flour and cornstarch.

2. Sugar:
- **Granulated Sugar:** Brown sugar, coconut sugar, honey, maple syrup, or agave nectar.
- **Powdered Sugar:** Blend granulated sugar with cornstarch in a food processor.

3. Butter:
- **Unsalted Butter:** Salted butter (adjust salt in the recipe), ghee, coconut oil, or vegetable shortening.
- **Oil:** Equal parts vegetable oil, olive oil, or coconut oil for melted butter.

4. Eggs:
- **Whole Eggs:** Unsweetened applesauce, mashed bananas, yogurt, or buttermilk.
- **Egg Whites:** Aquafaba (chickpea brine), flaxseed gel, or commercial egg replacers.

5. Milk:
- **Whole Milk:** Skim milk, 2% milk, almond milk, soy milk, or oat milk.
- **Buttermilk:** Mix regular milk with vinegar or lemon juice (1 cup milk + 1 tablespoon vinegar).

6. Cream:
- **Heavy Cream:** Greek yogurt, coconut cream, or evaporated milk.
- **Half-and-Half:** Equal parts whole milk and light cream.

7. Baking Powder:
- **Baking Powder:** Baking soda with an acidic ingredient (lemon juice, yogurt, buttermilk).

8. Tomato Sauce:

- **Tomato Sauce:** Crushed tomatoes blended with herbs or a jar of marinara sauce.
- **Tomato Paste:** Tomato sauce cooked down or blended sun-dried tomatoes.

9. Garlic:

- **Fresh Garlic:** Garlic powder or minced garlic from a jar.

10. Herbs (Fresh):

- **Basil:** Oregano, thyme, or parsley.
- **Cilantro:** Parsley, mint, or basil.
- **Rosemary:** Thyme, sage, or savory.

11. Cheese:

- **Cheddar:** Colby, Monterey Jack, or gouda.
- **Parmesan:** Pecorino Romano or Asiago.
- **Cream Cheese:** Greek yogurt or ricotta.

12. Nuts:

- **Almonds:** Walnuts, pecans, or hazelnuts.
- **Pine Nuts:** Sunflower seeds or chopped almonds.

13. Wine (Cooking):

- **White Wine:** Chicken or vegetable broth, or white grape juice.
- **Red Wine:** Beef or vegetable broth, grape juice, or balsamic vinegar.

14. Salt:

- **Table Salt:** Sea salt, kosher salt, or Himalayan pink salt.

30 DAYS

MEAL PLAN

	DAY 1
BREAKFAST:	Greek Yogurt Parfait
LUNCH:	Grilled Chicken Salad
SNACK:	Fresh Fruit
DINNER:	Baked Salmon, Quinoa, Broccoli

	DAY 2
BREAKFAST:	Oatmeal with Berries
LUNCH:	Quinoa and Black Bean Bowl
SNACK:	Mixed Nuts
DINNER:	Vegetable Stir-Fry, Brown Rice

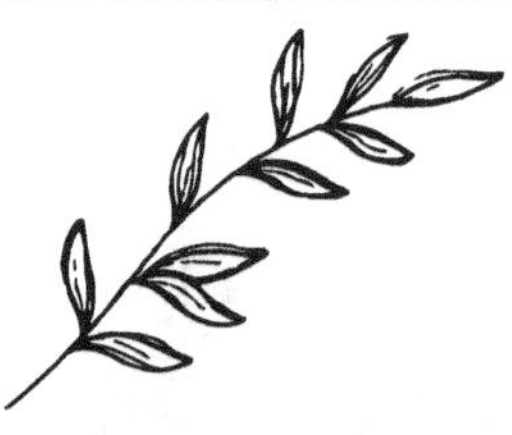 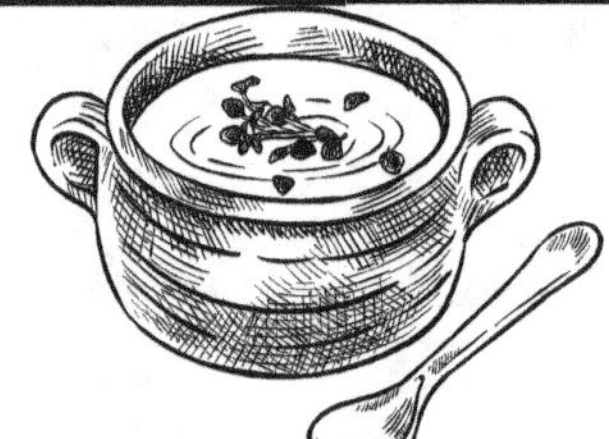 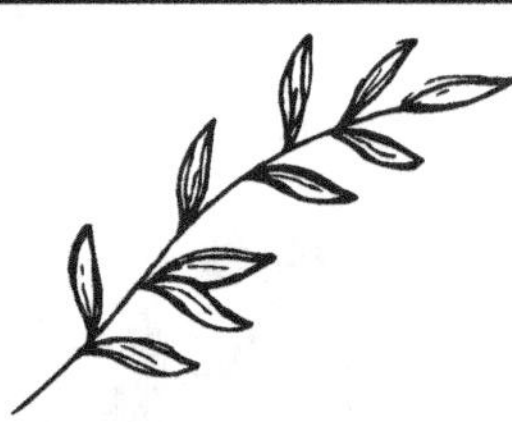

	DAY 3
BREAKFAST:	Scrambled Eggs, Avocado
LUNCH:	Chickpea Salad Wrap
SNACK:	Hummus with Veggies
DINNER:	Turkey Meatballs, Sweet Potato

	DAY 4
BREAKFAST:	Smoothie with Spinach
LUNCH:	Lentil Soup and Whole Grain Bread
SNACK:	Greek Yogurt with Berries
DINNER:	Grilled Shrimp, Couscous

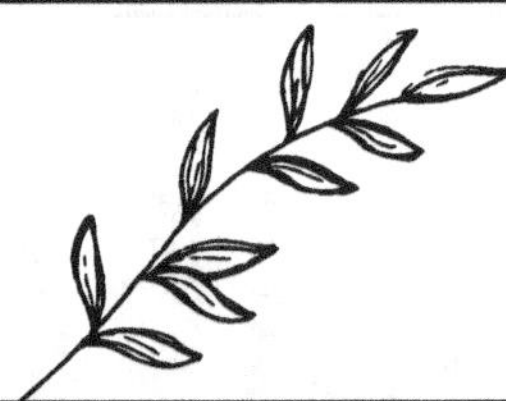 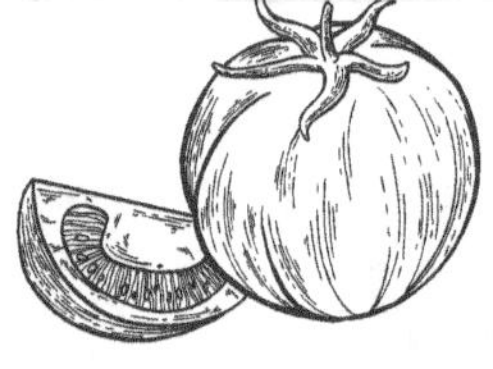 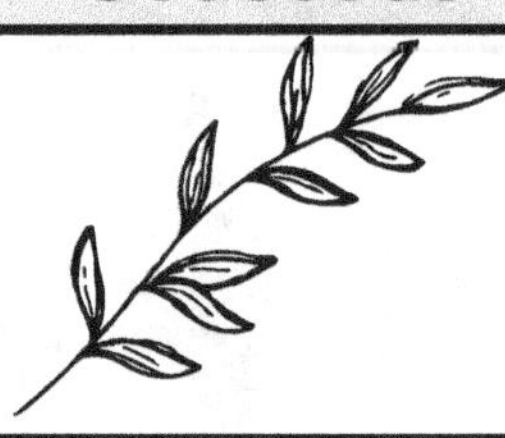

	DAY 5
BREAKFAST:	Whole Grain Toast, Peanut Butter
LUNCH:	Turkey and Veggie Wrap
SNACK:	Fresh Apple Slices
DINNER:	Chicken and Vegetable Skewers

	DAY 6
BREAKFAST:	Overnight Chia Pudding
LUNCH:	Quinoa Salad with Vinaigrette
SNACK:	Almond Butter with Celery
DINNER:	Baked Cod, Asparagus

DAY 7		DAY 8	
BREAKFAST:	Banana Walnut Muffins	**BREAKFAST:**	Spinach and Feta Omelette
LUNCH:	**Sweet Potato and Black Bean Bowl**	**LUNCH:**	Chicken Caesar Salad
SNACK:	Greek Yogurt with Granola	**SNACK:**	Cottage Cheese with Pineapple
DINNER:	Vegetarian Stir-Fried Tofu	**DINNER:**	Grilled Chicken, Quinoa, Broccoli

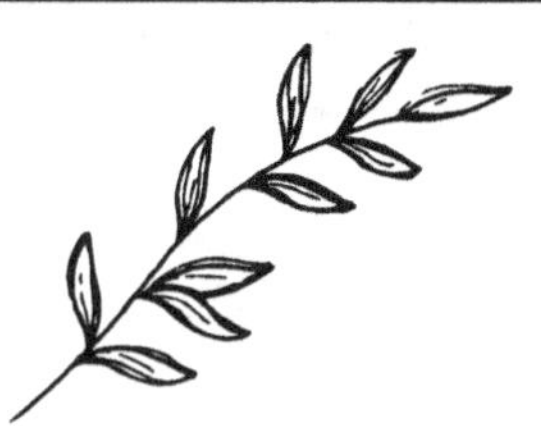
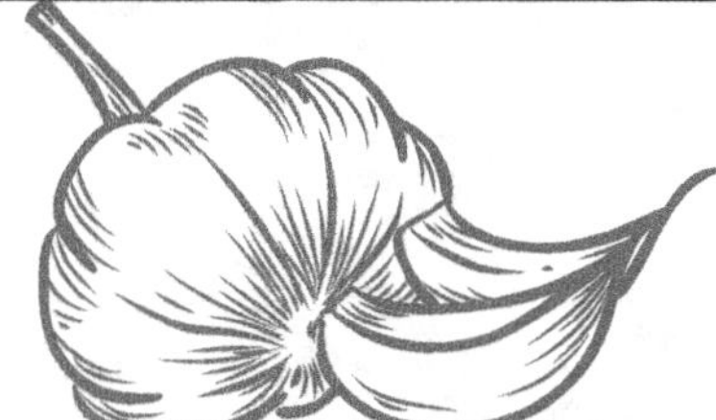

DAY 9		DAY 10	
BREAKFAST:	Acai Bowl with Granola	**BREAKFAST:**	Whole Grain Pancakes
LUNCH:	Veggie Wrap with Hummus	**LUNCH:**	Lentil Curry with Basmati Rice
SNACK:	Mixed Berries with Yogurt	**SNACK:**	Raw Veggies with Hummus
DINNER:	Baked Tilapia, Brown Rice	**DINNER:**	Beef Stir-Fry, Quinoa

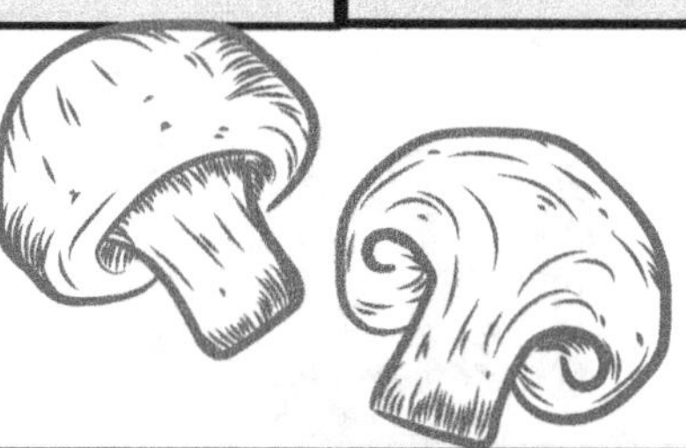

DAY 11		DAY 12	
BREAKFAST:	Avocado Toast with Egg	**BREAKFAST:**	Smoothie with Berries
LUNCH:	Mediterranean Quinoa Bowl	**LUNCH:**	Caprese Salad
SNACK:	Apple Slices with Almond Butter	**SNACK:**	Greek Yogurt with Walnuts
DINNER:	Turkey Chili with Cornbread	**DINNER:**	Grilled Salmon, Sweet Potato

DAY 13	DAY 14
BREAKFAST: Chia Seed Smoothie Bowl	**BREAKFAST:** Breakfast Burrito
LUNCH: Chickpea and Veggie Stir-Fry	**LUNCH:** Turkey and Avocado Wrap
SNACK: Fresh Fruit Salad	**SNACK:** Trail Mix
DINNER: Baked Chicken, Couscous	**DINNER:** Quinoa Stuffed Bell Peppers

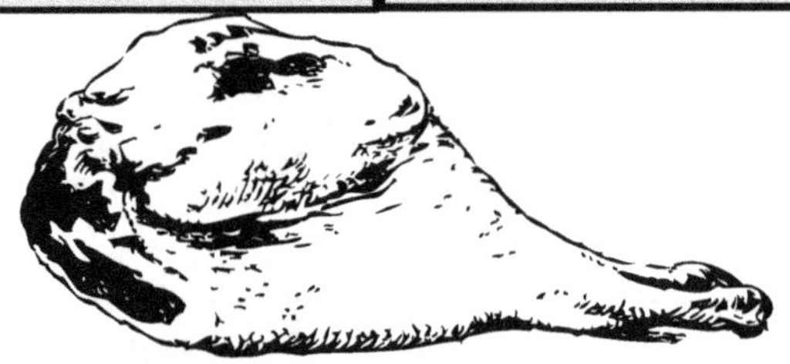

DAY 15	DAY 16
BREAKFAST: Yogurt Parfait with Granola	**BREAKFAST:** Vegetable Omelette
LUNCH: Quinoa Salad with Chickpeas	**LUNCH:** Lentil Soup and Whole Grain Bread
SNACK: Cottage Cheese with Berries	**SNACK:** Greek Yogurt with Mango
DINNER: Baked Cod, Brown Rice	**DINNER:** Grilled Shrimp, Quinoa

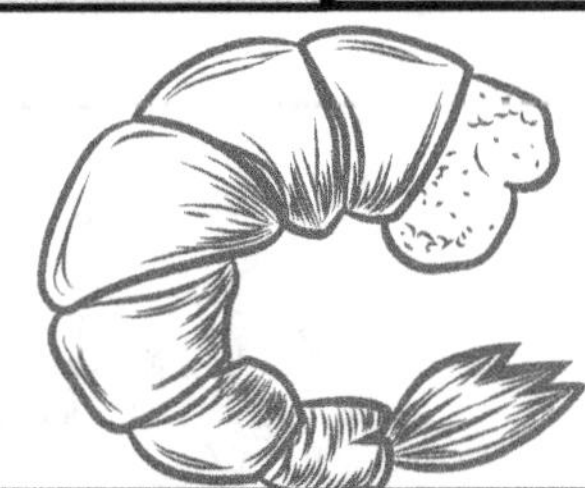

DAY 17	DAY 18
BREAKFAST: Peanut Butter Banana Toast	**BREAKFAST:** Blueberry Protein Pancakes
LUNCH: Turkey and Veggie Stir-Fry	**LUNCH:** Caprese Quinoa Bowl
SNACK: Fresh Apple Slices	**SNACK:** Almond Butter with Carrots
DINNER: Chicken Fajitas, Black Beans	**DINNER:** Baked Tilapia, Sweet Potato

DAY 19	
BREAKFAST: Smoothie Bowl with Kiwi	
LUNCH: Spinach and Feta Chickpea Salad	
SNACK: Mixed Nuts	
DINNER: Veggie Stir-Fried Tofu, Brown Rice	

DAY 20	
BREAKFAST: Breakfast Burrito Bowl	
LUNCH: Grilled Chicken Caesar Wrap	
SNACK: Hummus with Cucumber	
DINNER: Turkey Bolognese, Whole Wheat Pasta	

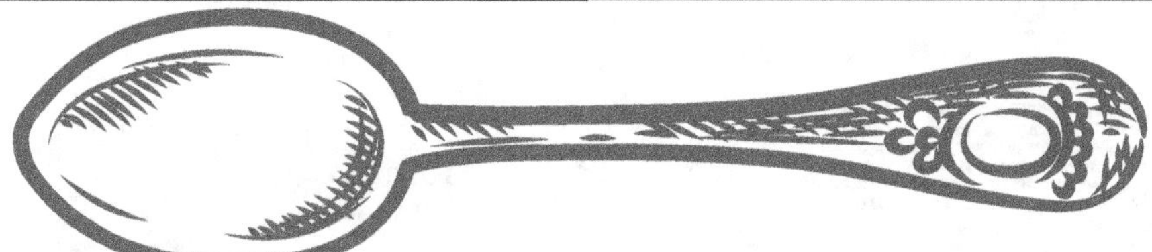

DAY 21	
BREAKFAST: Overnight Oats with Berries	
LUNCH: Quinoa and Black Bean Bowl	
SNACK: Greek Yogurt with Granola	
DINNER: Grilled Chicken, Quinoa, Broccoli	

DAY 22	
BREAKFAST: Acai Smoothie Bowl	
LUNCH: Chickpea Salad Wrap	
SNACK: Fresh Fruit Salad	
DINNER: Baked Cod, Asparagus	

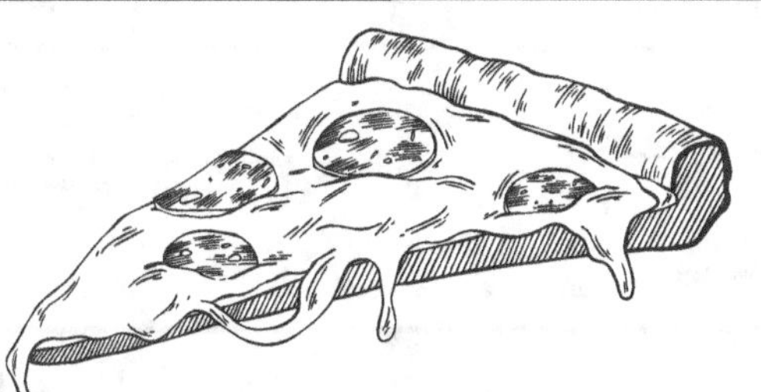

DAY 23	
BREAKFAST: Veggie Omelette	
LUNCH: Mediterranean Quinoa Bowl	
SNACK: Greek Yogurt with Walnuts	
DINNER: Grilled Shrimp, Sweet Potato	

DAY 24	
BREAKFAST: Chia Seed Pudding	
LUNCH: Lentil Curry with Basmati Rice	
SNACK: **Mixed Berries with Yogurt**	
DINNER: Turkey Chili with Cornbread	

DAY 25		DAY 26	
BREAKFAST:	Banana Walnut Muffins	**BREAKFAST:**	Oatmeal with Almond Butter
LUNCH:	Caprese Salad	**LUNCH:**	Veggie Stir-Fried Tofu
SNACK:	**Cottage Cheese with Pineapple**	**SNACK:**	Hummus with Veggies
DINNER:	Quinoa Stuffed Bell Peppers	**DINNER:**	Chicken and Vegetable Skewers

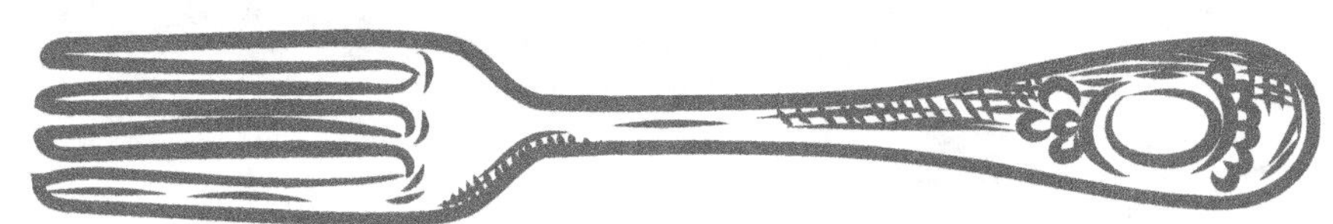

DAY 27		DAY 28	
BREAKFAST:	Smoothie with Spinach	**BREAKFAST:**	Whole Grain Pancakes
LUNCH:	Turkey and Avocado Wrap	**LUNCH:**	Quinoa Salad with Vinaigrette
SNACK:	Almond Butter with Celery	**SNACK:**	Trail Mix
DINNER:	Baked Salmon, Quinoa, Broccoli	**DINNER:**	Beef Stir-Fry, Brown Rice

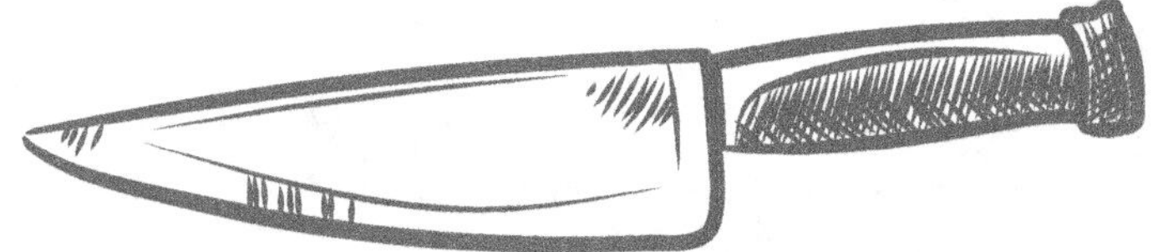

DAY 29		DAY 30	
BREAKFAST:	Avocado Toast with Egg	**BREAKFAST:**	Greek Yogurt Parfait
LUNCH:	Chickpea and Veggie Stir-Fry	**LUNCH:**	Quinoa and Black Bean Bowl
SNACK:	Greek Yogurt with Mango	**SNACK:**	Fresh Apple Slices
DINNER:	Grilled Chicken, Couscous	**DINNER:**	Baked Tilapia, Brown Rice